Crohn's Disease &

Ulcerative Colitis

Fred Saibil, MD

KEY PORTER BOOKS

Cataloguing in Publication Data

Saibil, Fredric G., 1942–
    Crohn's disease & ulcerative colitis

(Your personal health series)
Rev. ed.
ISBN 1-55013-819-7

1. Enteritis, Regional – Popular works.
2. Ulcerative colitis – Popular works.
I. Canadian Medical Association. II. Title.
III. Title: Crohn's disease and ulcerative colitis.
IV. Series.

RC862.I53S25 1996   616.3'44   C96-932121-X

The publisher gratefully acknowledges the assistance of the Canada
Council and the Ontario Arts Council.

Key Porter Books Limited
70 The Esplanade
Toronto, Ontario
Canada M5E 1R2

Diagrams: Martyn Lengden
Typesetting: Heidy Lawrance Associates

Distributed in the United States by Firefly Books
Printed and bound in Canada

2 3 4 5 04 03 02 01

Contents

Introduction / v

Chapter One: The Normal GI System and IBD / 1

Chapter Two: Who Gets IBD? What Causes It? / 9

Chapter Three: Symptoms and Signs / 19

Chapter Four: How Is IBD Diagnosed? / 29

Chapter Five: Diet and IBD / 37

Chapter Six: Drugs and IBD / 59

Chapter Seven: Surgery for IBD / 99

Chapter Eight: Children with IBD / 135

Chapter Nine: Complications of IBD / 139

Chapter Ten: Cancer and IBD / 159

Chapter Eleven: Living with IBD / 165

Chapter Twelve: Looking Ahead / 187

Table of Drug Names / 189

Glossary / 191

Further Resources / 200

Index / 203

Introduction

The term "inflammatory bowel disease" (IBD) refers to Crohn's disease and ulcerative colitis, two closely related conditions that cause persistent or recurring inflammation of one or more parts of the intestine. Crohn's disease is named after the late Dr. Burrill Crohn of New York, who was one of the first people to describe this disease in medical literature. Whereas Crohn's disease can affect any part of the gastrointestinal system, from the mouth to the anus, ulcerative colitis occurs only in the colon (large intestine).

Although these diseases are common, it is only in the past ten to fifteen years that it has become acceptable to talk about them publicly. Heart disease, diabetes, and even cancer have been freely discussed for many years, but no one wanted to hear about diarrhea, bloody bowel movements, or the need for frequent, urgent trips to the bathroom. The causes of these conditions are unknown. For years they were thought to be due to stress, but this is not the case. There is no known cure for Crohn's disease; ulcerative colitis can be cured, but only by surgical removal of the whole colon, including the rectum.

IBD can start at any age, but usually begins in the late teens or early adulthood or – less often – in middle age. Both Crohn's and ulcerative colitis are sometimes associated with a variety of medical problems outside of the intestine, including arthritis, skin conditions, kidney stones, cancer, and gallstones, among others.

Managing a chronic disease requires a team effort, and the team consists of the patient (and possibly the patient's family), the doctor (and possibly additional doctors), and sometimes other healthcare professionals. If patients are taught which problems they can treat (or at least start to treat) themselves, and which ones should be promptly reported, they achieve a greater degree of independence. For many patients, this means being able to go about their daily lives without worry.

This book, which is aimed primarily at patients and their families, provides a comprehensive review of IBD. Every effort has been made to avoid complex medical terminology. When such terms are necessary, definitions are provided in the text or in the glossary.

Topics covered include the signs, symptoms, and complications of IBD; nutritional issues, including lactose intolerance and other causes of gas and diarrhea; standard and newer drug treatments; surgery, with explanations of both minor and major operations; problems relating particularly to children with IBD; and various issues affecting everyday life, as well as self-help strategies for dealing with them.

Remember, this book is designed to educate you, not to frighten you. Having IBD can be difficult, but you can learn to live with it – and to fight back. This book will help you do that.

O N E

The Normal GI System and IBD

The Normal Gastrointestinal System

Learning about a medical subject is much like learning about anything else. You have to start with the basics and build on that. To learn about diseased bowel, you first have to learn about healthy bowel.

The bowel is part of the gastrointestinal system, commonly referred to as the gastrointestinal tract, or GI tract, for short. The GI tract begins at the mouth and ends with the anal canal. Most of it lies in the abdominal cavity, which is lined with a thin, transparent tissue called the *peritoneum*. The chief function of the GI tract is to digest food – break it down into usable materials, then absorb them and eliminate the waste products.

When you eat, food goes from your *mouth* down your *esophagus* (the swallowing tube), into your *stomach*. Your stomach grinds the food and dilutes it. The resulting semiliquid gradually empties into the *small bowel*, or small intestine, which is 20 feet (6 meters) long and lies coiled in the middle of your abdomen.

The small bowel is made up of three parts. The first is the *duodenum*, which is just a few inches (centimeters) long. The

The Gastrointestinal Tract

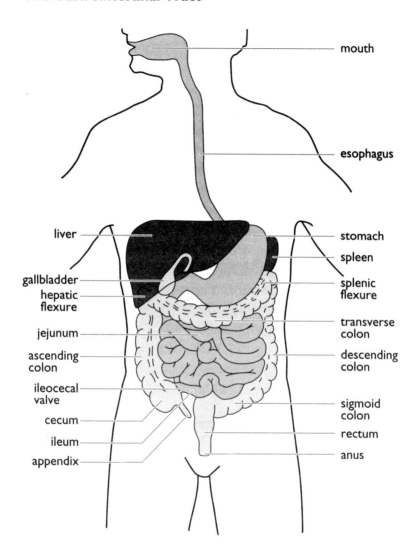

next part, about 10 feet (3 meters) long, is the *jejunum*. This is where most of the food that we eat is digested and absorbed. The last 10 feet of the small bowel is the *ileum*. The juices produced by all three parts of the small intestine, as well as juices from the liver, gallbladder, and pancreas, digest (break down) food and convert it into usable elements. Most carbohydrates (e.g., breads, potatoes, and pasta) and proteins (e.g., meat, eggs, fish) are broken down and absorbed in the jejunum. Fats (e.g., butter, oil, margarine) are digested more slowly and require both the jejunum and ileum to be absorbed. Two things are absorbed exclusively by the ileum: vitamin B_{12} and bile salts. This point becomes important when people undergo surgery to remove this part of the small bowel.

The ileum runs into the *colon*, low down on the right side of the abdomen. At the junction of the ileum and colon is a muscular thickening known as the *ileocecal valve*. It is not really a valve, but it opens and closes like a valve. This permits the small bowel to discharge its contents (mainly waste products) intermittently into the colon.

The colon, also known as the large bowel or large intestine, is much wider than the small intestine and is about 5 feet (1.5 meters) long. It too has different sections. The first is the *cecum*, which is a little cul-de-sac that lies below the junction of the ileum and the colon. The cecum probably does not have any specific function but is a remnant of evolution. The same may be true for the *appendix*, which projects from the cecum, although the appendix contains a lot of lymphoid tissue (part of the immune system) and this may be important.

Running upward from the cecum is the *ascending colon*. As you follow it, you will come to a sharp bend called the *hepatic flexure*. "Flexure" means "bend"; "hepatic" (from the Greek word "hepar", "liver") indicates that the bend is at the liver.

The segment of colon that runs from the hepatic flexure

across the abdomen is called the *transverse colon*. The colon then turns sharply again at the *splenic flexure* (at the spleen).

The segment of colon that runs downward from the splenic flexure is called the *descending colon*. Following the descending colon is the *sigmoid colon*, named after the Greek letter *sigma* ("s") because the sigmoid curves frequently.

The *rectum* makes up the last section of the colon, although it is often treated as a separate entity. The *anal canal* is the outlet for the rectum. It is surrounded by the anal sphincter, a valvelike muscle that controls the passage of stool (waste matter) out of the rectum. The *anus* is the opening at the end of the canal.

These different sections of the colon do not have distinctive functions. The terms for the various sections of the colon allow doctors to communicate more precisely with other doctors when describing a problem.

The colon has two main functions. One is to store waste material. The other is to absorb salt and water.

The terms "stool" and "feces" (pronounced fee-sees) refer to the material discharged from the rectum, whether it is solid or liquid. When the stool starts out near the cecum, it is brown water – it looks just like a polluted river! When the stool comes out of the rectum, it is supposed to be a nice, neat package – not too hard, not too soft, not too big, not too small – several inches long and sausage-shaped. As the brown fluid moves around the colon, the water is gradually absorbed by the lining of the colon so that the stool becomes more and more solid.

About 75 percent of a normal stool in the rectum is water. The GI tract is full of millions of different germs, mainly bacteria, mostly in the colon. They have a short life span and are constantly dying and being replaced by newly born bacteria; live and dead bacteria contribute about 8 percent to the bulk of the stool. About 4 percent comes from undigested food roughage (fiber). The lining of the whole GI tract replaces itself approximately every 72 hours, which means that a layer of dead tissue regularly "peels off"; this makes up about 3 percent of stool. The colon is always producing mucus, which is nature's lubricant, and this also ends up in the stool (1 percent). The remaining 9 percent is composed of a variety of substances.

When your rectum fills with stool, a message is sent to your brain telling it that the rectum needs to be emptied. If you sit on the toilet, the rectum will contract (squeeze), the anal sphincter will open, and the stool will be pushed out through the anal canal into the toilet. The normal process of digestion will have been completed.

Inflammatory Bowel Disease (IBD)

Inflammation – the word means "being set on fire" – is a localized protective response that occurs when tissue is damaged or destroyed. Its purpose is to wall off, dilute, or destroy an injurious agent. Acute inflammation is characterized by pain, heat, redness, and swelling. Chronic inflammation is a less dramatic process. It may proceed without any of these features, yet it results in distortion, and sometimes destruction, of tissues, often leading to permanent scarring.

Inflammatory bowel disease is just that – disease in which the bowel becomes inflamed. By convention the term refers to just two diseases: ulcerative colitis (UC) and Crohn's disease (CD).

Both UC and CD probably first appeared as isolated cases several centuries ago, but they did not attract medical interest until the last half of the 19th century. Ulcerative colitis was described and named in 1875 in a medical textbook published in London, England. In 1913, an article in a British journal mentioned a group of patients with what was probably Crohn's disease. But it wasn't until a more widely publicized report was published in the United States in 1932 by Dr. Crohn and his

It is common for different doctors to make up new names for specific diseases, especially those of unknown cause. Sometimes multiple names occur because what were thought to be two separate diseases turn out to be one and the same. For example, Crohn's disease was originally thought to occur only in the small intestine, and not in the colon.

Other Names for Ulcerative Colitis and Crohn's Disease

Ulcerative colitis (UC)
- idiopathic ulcerative colitis (idiopathic means "of unknown cause")
- nonspecific ulcerative colitis

Crohn's disease (CD)
- ileitis, terminal ileitis ("terminal" refers to the terminus, "end" of the ileum)
- regional enteritis, regional ileitis
- granulomatous ileitis/enteritis/colitis ("granulomatous" refers to a specific appearance under the microscope)
- Crohn's disease of the colon/ileum/jejunum/duodenum/stomach

colleagues that the disease came to be known as Crohn's disease.

One Disease, Two, or More?

Some experts in the field have thought that ulcerative colitis and Crohn's disease are merely two forms of the same disease, perhaps because some people who "clearly" have ulcerative colitis "clearly" develop features of Crohn's disease at a later date. It is extremely rare, though, for an expert to diagnose Crohn's colitis, and then change the diagnosis later to ulcerative colitis. It is also extremely rare for both diseases to coexist in one person.

Because we cannot always tell if the problem is ulcerative colitis or Crohn's disease, we tell some patients that they have "indeterminate colitis." This too has encouraged the perception of IBD as just one disease. In many cases, not being able to say which kind of colitis it is doesn't matter. Except when surgery is necessary, most treatments are the same for both ulcerative colitis and Crohn's disease.

Where Does Ulcerative Colitis Occur?

Ulcerative colitis occurs only in the colon. It always involves the rectum. It should be continuous – that is, not confined to patches.

Some patients have inflammation just in the rectum (known as ulcerative proctitis). Others have it in the rectum and the sigmoid colon. Some have it in the rectum, the sigmoid colon, and the descending colon up to the splenic flexure. Others have it from the rectum around into the transverse colon. Some have it as far as the hepatic flexure. Yet others have it throughout the entire colon to the cecum.

Ulcerative colitis involves the rectum plus or minus the sigmoid in 30 percent of cases, approximately the left half to two-thirds of the colon in 40 percent of cases, and the whole colon in 30 percent of cases.

Learning about medicine means accepting the fact that we can never say "never" and we can never say "always." Occasionally there are patients in whom ulcerative colitis is not continuous. What we see then is involvement of the rectum and part of the descending colon, plus a patch in the cecum, usually around the opening into the appendix. The patch near the appendix looks just like ulcerative colitis anywhere else. As you will see, patchy disease is typical of Crohn's disease; however, it is believed that these people with a patch of colitis around the appendix and typical ulcerative colitis elsewhere do in fact have ulcerative colitis.

In some patients with ulcerative colitis, the inner lining of the last few inches (centimeters) of the ileum becomes mildly inflamed. This inflammation is called backwash ileitis; it does not cause any symptoms or problems. We don't know why some patients get backwash ileitis and others don't.

Exactly What Is Inflamed in Ulcerative Colitis?

In ulcerative colitis, inflammation is usually confined to the inner lining of the colon, or *mucosa*. The surface of this inner lining becomes raw and bleeds easily, and looks a lot like scraped skin.

Where Does Crohn's Disease Occur?

Crohn's disease can occur anywhere from the mouth to the anus. Most commonly (45 percent) it occurs in the end of the ileum and the beginning of the colon (cecum plus or minus ascending colon). Next most commonly (35 percent) it occurs just in the end of the ileum. Third most commonly (20 percent) it occurs just in the colon. Here it may be patchy or continuous, and may or may not involve the rectum. In a few patients the jejunum, duodenum, stomach, or esophagus is involved. For most patients with inflammation in these areas, the ileum or the colon or both are involved as well, but in a few people the disease is isolated in one of those locations. When Crohn's disease occurs in the mouth, it is almost always associated with Crohn's disease elsewhere in the GI tract.

Exactly What Is Inflamed in Crohn's Disease?

In Crohn's disease, the entire thickness of the bowel wall, from the inner lining (the mucosa) through the muscle layers to the outer lining (the *serosa*), is inflamed. In addition to swelling of the bowel wall, Crohn's disease causes swelling of the *mesentery*, a fan-shaped piece of tissue that connects the small intestine to the back wall of the abdomen and contains the main intestinal blood vessels and lymph glands.

TWO

Who Gets IBD? What Causes It?

Who Gets IBD?

Inflammatory bowel disease can begin at any age. Most commonly it appears between the ages of 15 and 30 or – less often – between the ages of 45 and 60. It occurs throughout the world, but it is much more prevalent in temperate climates than in tropical ones. It is found more often in developed countries such as those in North America, Scandinavia, and Western Europe. Most studies report that IBD is more likely to occur in people of a higher socioeconomic bracket. However, poorer people are less likely to seek treatment for their disease, so this may skew the studies.

Is IBD More Common in Certain Ethnic Groups?

IBD is three times as common in Jews as in non-Jews. But this applies only to Ashkenazi Jews, who are mostly from Eastern Europe – not to Sephardic Jews, who come from Spain and other Mediterranean countries, or to Asiatic Jews. It is much less common in blacks and Asians than in Caucasians. There is some evidence that Orientals are unlikely to have IBD if they live in the Far East, but develop it more frequently if they move to North America.

Men and women seem to get ulcerative colitis in equal

numbers, but Crohn's disease is more common in women than in men.

How Common Is IBD?
Many studies have been done to estimate the frequency of inflammatory bowel disease. Estimates in North America range from 10 per 100,000 to 1,000 per 100,000.

Is IBD Increasing?
Statistics for ulcerative colitis have not changed significantly of late, but Crohn's disease has been on the increase. Part of the reason is a change in medical thinking about IBD. It was originally thought that Crohn's disease occurred only in the small intestine, while all chronic colitis was ulcerative colitis. In the 1950s someone wrote an article asserting that Crohn's disease could occur in the colon, though it was very uncommon. The occasional case of Crohn's colitis was then diagnosed over the next few years. In the late 1960s Crohn's disease of the colon was found to be quite common. Many patients who had originally been told that they had ulcerative colitis were told, "You never had ulcerative colitis. It was Crohn's disease from the start, but we didn't know it at the time."

What Causes IBD?
We know a lot about IBD, but we don't yet know what causes it. Here are some of the factors that may play a role.

Genes May Predispose You to IBD.
There are several reasons for believing that IBD has a genetic component. If a person has ulcerative colitis, there is about a 10 percent chance of IBD in other members of the extended family, with ulcerative colitis more likely than Crohn's disease. On the other hand, if a person has Crohn's disease, there is a

25 to 30 percent chance of IBD in the extended family, with Crohn's disease more likely than ulcerative colitis. If a person has IBD, the risk of that person's child developing IBD is thought to be about 5 percent. It is important to recognize that this means that the child has about a 95 percent chance of *not* developing IBD. However, if both parents have IBD, the risk of IBD occurring in the children seems to be at least 50 percent.

Studies of identical twins have shown that if one twin develops Crohn's disease, the other twin will likely also develop it, usually within a few years. If one twin develops ulcerative colitis, however, the probability that the other member will develop ulcerative colitis is much less. There are no reports of one identical twin having ulcerative colitis and the other having Crohn's disease.

As well, researchers have identified a group of antibodies known as *antineutrophil cytoplasmic antibodies* (ANCA) which are present in high levels in patients with ulcerative colitis, and in a significant number of their relatives, even when those relatives do not have IBD. These antibodies are found in low levels in some patients with Crohn's disease and a small proportion of their relatives, and not at all in healthy families.

Certain diseases occur more commonly in patients with IBD. One of the best-known examples is the arthritic disease ankylosing spondylitis (see Chapter 9). Another example is cystic fibrosis, which is known to be a genetically transmitted disease. Several years ago, researchers showed that there was an association between multiple sclerosis and Crohn's disease, and it has been known for some time that people with Crohn's disease have a greater chance of having psoriasis. Associations such as these support the concept of a genetic predisposition to IBD.

Thus far, genetic techniques have not revealed any of the secrets of IBD. However, the science of identifying human

---

What about Stress?

The issue of stress and the gut is an important one. Many people in the general population (i.e., people who do not have IBD) have gastrointestinal problems when they are under stress, and this has led to an assumption that stress has a role to play in IBD as well. The condition known as irritable bowel syndrome (IBS) is a disorder in which people tend to have abdominal pain and irregular bowel movements without any intestinal inflammation. Many people with IBS have a considerable increase in their symptoms when they are mentally stressed. Everyone is familiar with the term "tension headaches," and people are not embarrassed to talk about them. But you don't hear a lot of people talking about their "tension vomiting" or "tension diarrhea" or "tension bellyaches," although these are every bit as common. As with tension headaches, tension gut symptoms can occur in any pattern, from occasionally to daily.

Doctors used to think that IBD was caused by stress. There is no evidence for this, and it is no longer believed by experts in the field. Controversy still exists, however, about the possible role of stress as a precipitating factor in flare-ups in a person with pre-existing IBD. Even if stress is a factor, it generally cannot be avoided, and the thought that a particular stress may cause a flare-up of the disease is in itself stressful.

People with IBD can also have IBS, and no doubt the occurrence of both conditions in the same person helps to perpetuate the idea that stress causes IBD. The experienced doctor and the experienced IBD patient know that IBD can begin when things are going well or when they are going badly. Saying that IBD is a psychological illness suggests that, because of the kind of person you are, you are in some way responsible for the disease. This is likely to make you feel guilty, which can make you feel even worse. Remember, it's not your fault!

---

genes is still in its early stages, and it is reasonable to expect positive results sometime in the future.

IBD and Infections

There is no convincing evidence that IBD is due to infection. But infectious colitis (which is caused by bacteria, viruses, or parasites) and ulcerative colitis are similar, and Crohn's disease is strikingly like intestinal tuberculosis (which is caused by a bacterium). Studies continue in this area and may provide some kind of clue to the cause of IBD.

Abnormal Immunity May Be a Factor.

Chapter 1 outlined the digestive functions of the GI tract. A second function, less well understood, is that of protecting the body against potentially harmful infectious agents or chemical substances.

The inner lining of the intestine (the mucosa) contains many types of immune cells that act as defenders in recognizing foreign substances, known as antigens. These cells prevent such substances from passing through the mucosa and entering the body. Some of these cells engulf the potentially harmful substances. Such cells are named "macrophages." Other cells, named "lymphocytes," produce antibodies, which are chemical products that bind to and inactivate foreign substances and infectious agents.

Sometimes this immune response in the mucosa breaks down and harmful agents or chemicals penetrate into the deeper layers of the intestine. This produces inflammation.

As well, researchers have shown that healthy people have an invisible intestinal "barrier" capable of preventing various substances from being absorbed into the intestinal wall. Canadian researchers have shown that this barrier is "leaky" in people with Crohn's disease. This means that substances that would not normally be absorbed may enter the intestinal tissues and trigger inflammation.

Numerous researchers have tried to show that IBD is an "autoimmune" disease, meaning that the disease occurs because the body attacks itself. The idea is based on the concept of molecular mimicry. The proposed scenario is as follows. A microbe attacks the intestine and the intestine produces antibodies. The antibodies get rid of the microbe. However, the antibodies are chemically so similar to the microbe that the body can't distinguish between the two. The body continues to react against the antibodies and this becomes a self-perpetuating inflammatory response. Multiple abnormalities of the immune system have in fact been detected in people with IBD, but many researchers think that these abnormalities are the *result* of the disease, not the cause. Even if these abnormalities perpetuate the disease, the initiating factor is the vital unknown.

A Blood-Vessel Abnormality May Cause Crohn's Disease.
An old idea, which has recently received renewed attention, is that Crohn's disease is due to an inadequate supply of oxygen to one or more parts of the intestine as a result of inflammation and blockage of small blood vessels within the intestine. Experimental studies interfering with blood flow create an appearance that is somewhat similar to Crohn's disease, with areas of inflammation and narrowing of the intestine.

A research group in London, England, believes that Crohn's disease is due to a chronic blood-vessel inflammation in reaction to a persistent infection with the measles virus within the inner lining of the blood vessels.

The work is very interesting, but it should be noted that countries where measles infections are severe and vaccination is rare have low rates of Crohn's disease.

Smoking Increases the Risk of Getting Crohn's Disease.
Numerous studies conducted since 1987 have demonstrated that cigarette smoking is a risk factor for Crohn's disease. A recent study has suggested that smoking also increases the likelihood that Crohn's disease will recur after surgery; giving up smoking soon after surgery makes a recurrence less likely. How smoking exerts these effects is unknown. However, the evidence is compelling enough that if you have Crohn's disease and you smoke, you should give it up. Paradoxically, nicotine seems to protect some people against ulcerative colitis!

As for second-hand smoke, a recent American study has shown that passive smoking carries an increased risk of IBD in children. This makes sense in Crohn's disease, which is associated with smoking, but goes contrary to what has been established in ulcerative colitis, where smoking should be protective.

Oral Contraceptives and IBD

Research on IBD among oral-contraceptive users is inconclusive. While the risk of developing IBD seems to be increased, stopping the pill often makes no difference.

Many gastroenterologists (physicians who specialize in treating diseases of the GI tract) consider it worthwhile for women with poorly controlled IBD to stop the pill temporarily to see what happens. If this is not possible, switching to a lower-estrogen pill is an alternative. Because the oral contraceptive remains the most effective form of birth control, women should carefully consider the potential benefits and risks of stopping the pill or avoiding it altogether.

Ulcerative Colitis As a Result of "Malnutrition" of the Colonic Mucosa (Inner Lining)

Within the past few years we've learned that compounds known as short-chain fatty acids are essential nutrients for the mucosa of the colon. These compounds are produced as bacteria break down complex carbohydrate residue (i.e., fiber) in the colon (see Chapter 1). If the colon is deprived of these compounds, the mucosa (inner lining) becomes inflamed and bleeds easily.

A European researcher named Roediger has suggested that ulcerative colitis is a nutritional deficiency disease of the colon in which there is an inadequate supply and/or delivery of short-chain fatty acids to the mucosa. He has treated some ulcerative colitis patients with short-chain fatty-acid enemas and has reported favorable results. Studies in the U.S. and Canada have demonstrated some benefit, but the results have not been dramatic. More recent research by other groups has not supported the hypothesis that UC is caused by a lack of short-chain fatty acids, despite the fact that selected patients do seem to respond to this treatment.

Odds and Ends

Within the past ten years, a growing body of experimental and clinical evidence has suggested that a class of chemicals known as reactive oxygen metabolites may play an important role in the development of IBD. Some of these chemicals are classified as "oxidants"; others are referred to as "free radicals." Some of the drug therapies used in IBD, such as 5-ASA (see Chapter 6), have potent antioxidant activity. However, much more work needs to be done to determine the role of these chemicals.

- Many scientists have stated that nitric oxide is the chemical of the nineties. This small molecule has only recently been discovered to be an important chemical in many disease processes in the body. Studies are under way to determine if this fascinating substance plays any role in IBD.
- Patients with ulcerative colitis are much less likely than are members of a comparable control group to have undergone an appendectomy. It has been suggested that appendectomy protects against UC. However, it is also possible that something about the colon or appendix in patients with UC makes appendicitis less likely. More study is needed.
- From time to time, researchers have tried to link dietary factors to the development of IBD. Milk, corn flakes, a

high intake of refined sugar, baker's yeast, and various other dietary constituents have been put forward as risk factors. To date, these theories either have been disproved or have not been conclusively proved.

- In recent years, some researchers have tried to tie the risk of IBD to a higher number of childhood infections. Other researchers have said just the opposite, citing improved sanitation in developed countries, where IBD is much more common.

So Where Does This Leave Us?

Our current understanding of the development of IBD is as follows. First, you must have a genetically susceptible subject. This person must then come in contact with some agent or substance that, through some defect in the normal intestinal defense system, is able to penetrate the intestinal wall. This sets up an inflammatory response. A defect in regulating the inflammatory response must also exist so that, once the immune system is activated, a complex process is started that the body is unable to stop.

We still have no answer to the question of what causes IBD, but research is ongoing. There is every reason to be optimistic and believe that the causes of ulcerative colitis and Crohn's disease will eventually be found.

THREE

Symptoms and Signs

ymptoms are things that you can *feel* and tell your doctor about. Pain, poor appetite, nausea, and diarrhea are common symptoms of IBD. Signs are things that you or your doctor can *observe*. Being pale, having a rash, or passing blood into the toilet are all common signs of IBD. At times symptoms and signs are difficult to separate. If you have an itchy rash, the itch is a symptom and the rash is a sign. A diagnosis is easier to make with both symptoms and signs. This is why your doctor will frequently ask you many questions about a complaint. The more information you give, the more accurate the diagnosis will be, and the better the treatment.

Symptoms and Signs of Ulcerative Colitis

The most typical characteristic of ulcerative colitis is bloody diarrhea; bloody diarrhea makes us think of ulcerative colitis and ulcerative colitis makes us think of bloody diarrhea. There are always exceptions, of course. Some people with this condition have bleeding without diarrhea and some even have bleeding with constipation (particularly people with ulcerative proctitis). Mostly, though, it's bloody diarrhea.

Next to that, the most typical symptom of ulcerative colitis is the false urge: you get a feeling that you are going to have a bowel movement, but when you get to the toilet nothing or almost nothing comes out. Sometimes there's some gas, or some "wet" gas, or a little blood, or even a bit of stool, but there is no reasonable amount of stool. The total number of trips to the toilet, for actual bowel movements and false urges combined, is one of the indicators of how severe an attack of colitis is.

As a *rough* guide, 2 to 5 trips to the toilet in 24 hours indicate a mild attack of colitis, 5 to 10 trips indicate a moderate attack, and 10 to 20 or 30 trips indicate a severe attack.

Closely related to the false urge is a symptom named *tenesmus*. You experience it as persistent pressure in the region of the anus; it feels like a constant false urge. It is usually not relieved completely (sometimes not at all) by passing gas or fluid or even stool.

Tenesmus is typically due to inflammation and spasm of the rectum. When a normal rectum is filled with stool, it sends a message to the brain that says, "Go to the bathroom and have a bowel movement." A healthy person responds by going to the bathroom, but can also have the brain say to the rectum, "Not now – I'm busy." The rectum will relax and the urge to go the bathroom will disappear. When the rectum is inflamed, however, it is in spasm all the time. A rectum in spasm sends the same message to the brain as a full rectum. You constantly feel you need to go to the bathroom. The rectum does not accept the message "Not now – I'm busy." Even when you sit on the toilet, even if you have a bowel movement, this urge to pass stool is not completely relieved. The reason, of course, is that the rectum is still inflamed and therefore still in spasm, so the message from the rectum to the brain doesn't change very much.

Aside from bloody stools and frequent trips to the toilet, many people with ulcerative colitis experience crampy pain in the abdomen, low down on the left side, across the lower abdomen, or across the upper and lower abdomen. Such pain, often described as squeezing in nature, is usually followed by a trip to the toilet. Typically, the pain is relieved by passing stool or gas, or both.

Other symptoms that may be experienced by people with ulcerative colitis are reduced appetite, weight loss, fever, chills, and sweats. These symptoms are either absent or mild in a patient with a mild attack of colitis, but can be dramatic in a severe attack.

Are People with Ulcerative Colitis Sick All the Time?

It is important to recognize that most people with ulcerative colitis are well between attacks. In any given patient, attacks, or flare-ups, may occur frequently (every few weeks) or rarely (every few years). A person may have multiple flare-ups one year and then none for several years, or any other irregular pattern that you can imagine. The average risk of a flare-up is about 10 percent per year. A small number of people with ulcerative colitis (about 5 percent) have what is known as chronic continuous colitis.

Signs of Ulcerative Colitis

For most patients with ulcerative colitis there are few signs of the disease, other than blood in the stool. In some patients, the doctor can feel a fullness in the right lower quadrant of the abdomen. This is because the stool piles up in the ascending colon during an attack. The colon is extremely inefficient at emptying itself when it is inflamed, even though you may go to the bathroom many times.

Symptoms of Crohn's Disease

Crohn's disease is somewhat more complicated than ulcerative colitis because it can affect different parts of the GI tract. The general symptoms are crampy abdominal pain, diarrhea, and weight loss. Pain is most often felt around the navel and/or lower right part of the abdomen. It is often associated with eating, and can begin during a meal, soon after, or within an hour or so. A steady, dull ache in the lower right abdomen may also be felt. It is usually somewhat worse with activity, especially anything that jiggles the abdomen, such as jogging. Crohn's patients also suffer from fatigue and poor appetite.

Symptoms of Small-Bowel Crohn's Disease

Some 70 to 80 percent of patients with small-bowel Crohn's disease complain of crampy abdominal pain, diarrhea, and weight loss. Many patients quickly learn that they can avoid pain by avoiding food, and this is the main reason people lose weight. Occasionally a patient with small-bowel Crohn's is troubled by constipation rather than diarrhea.

IBD Lookalikes

Many other medical conditions are characterized by diarrhea and crampy pain, like inflammatory bowel disease. Diagnosing IBD means ruling them out.

- Infections can mimic IBD: food poisoning, traveler's diarrhea, antibiotic-associated colitis, gay bowel disease, yersiniosis, giardiasis, intestinal tuberculosis.
- Irritable bowel syndrome (IBS) can resemble Crohn's disease.
- Foods can cause chronic diarrhea: lactose, if you are lactose intolerant; caffeine; fructose; sorbitol, mannitol, xylitol; a high-fiber diet.
- Drugs can cause chronic diarrhea: antibiotics, nonsteroidal anti-inflammatory drugs (NSAIDs), 5-aminosalicylate, gold injections (for rheumatoid arthritis), methyldopa (for high blood pressure), and many others.
- Other IBD lookalikes include radiation enteritis after radiation treatment for certain cancers, ischemic (lack of blood flow) disease of the intestine, collagenous colitis.

"They thought I had appendicitis."

Some patients with undiagnosed small-bowel Crohn's become ill suddenly and go to the hospital with severe abdominal pain. The attack is similar to acute appendicitis, and surgery may be necessary to make the correct diagnosis. The appendix is usually removed, whether it is normal or not. This is a good idea for the most part, because any future attacks will not be blamed on appendicitis.

Is It Crohn's or Is It IBS?

The main alternative diagnosis to Crohn's disease is irritable bowel syndrome (IBS). However, people with IBS rarely lose weight. Early in the onset of symptoms of Crohn's disease there may not be weight loss, and this may delay the correct diagnosis. Here's a case in point.

A 21-year-old woman developed crampy pain around her navel and mild diarrhea with three to four mushy bowel movements a day. The crampy pain and diarrhea came mainly after meals. She was otherwise well and had never been sick before. She thought she might have "the flu." When the symptoms persisted for two weeks and became slightly worse, she went to see her family doctor. He examined her abdomen, said it was normal, and told her she probably had irritable bowel syndrome. No X-rays or blood tests were performed. The patient was reassured that nothing serious was wrong and was told there was nothing to be done for these mild symptoms.

Four weeks later the symptoms were still present and somewhat worse. The woman was now having four to six bowel movements a day, and occasionally got up at night to have them. She had lost ten pounds (almost five kilograms). She decided to go see her mother's family doctor. The physical examination, blood tests, and an X-ray of the colon were normal. Again she was told that she probably had irritable bowel syndrome. When asked if she was nervous, she said that she was. (Anyone having cramps in the abdomen and unpredictable diarrhea for six weeks is bound to be a little nervous!) She was offered a tranquilizer. She tried it, but it just made her feel dopey and did not change her symptoms.

Four more weeks passed. By this time she had lost 20 pounds. She went back to her own doctor. He arranged for a small-bowel X-ray which revealed Crohn's disease in the ileum. The woman was promptly referred to a gastroenterologist and treatment was started, with good results.

In the past, this was a very common sequence of events. Statistics in the 1970s indicated that the average time it took, from the point when someone began complaining until the diagnosis of Crohn's disease was made, was 3 years. Since some people were diagnosed quickly, this means that in other people the delay was much longer. Over the past 20 years, much more attention has been given to IBD in medical schools. As a result, doctors now think of it sooner, make the diagnosis more quickly, and start treatment faster. In many cases, this prevents the person from losing a lot of weight and becoming seriously ill.

Symptoms of Crohn's Disease of the Colon (Crohn's Colitis)
The symptoms of Crohn's colitis are variable, depending on whether the disease occurs in the right side of the colon, the left side, or the whole colon, and whether the rectum is involved. If the disease is primarily on the right side, you will have mainly cramps and diarrhea. If the disease is primarily on the left side or involves most of the colon, you will likely have cramps, diarrhea, and some blood in the stool. If the rectum is involved, you will have symptoms similar to ulcerative colitis, with false urges (see symptoms of ulcerative colitis in this chapter).

Symptoms of Crohn's Disease of the Ileum and Colon
If you have both small-bowel and large-bowel disease, you may experience symptoms of the disease from one location, the other, or both. Crohn's of the ileum can flare up when the colonic disease is quiet, and vice versa.

Symptoms of Crohn's Disease of the Stomach and/or Duodenum
Many people with Crohn's disease in this part of the GI system have no symptoms, and the inflammation is discovered by chance. Of those who do have symptoms, over 90 percent have pain or discomfort in the upper abdomen (right side, middle, or left side) that comes on during and soon after meals. Nausea, vomiting, or both occur in about 30 percent of patients. Weight loss occurs in over 50 percent of people with symptoms as a result of the tendency to eat less in order to avoid the symptoms. Occasionally, Crohn's disease of the duodenum will mimic ordinary duodenal ulcer disease. In this situation, pain is more likely to occur when you have not eaten for a few hours, and the pain will be relieved by food.

In some patients, Crohn's disease of the stomach and/or duodenum produces enough scarring that the outlet of the stomach into the duodenum becomes progressively narrower. The patient will complain of not being able to eat a normal-sized meal, a prolonged full or bloated feeling in the upper abdomen after meals, nausea, and, often, a decrease in appetite.

Symptoms of Crohn's Disease of the Esophagus
This is so rare a form of Crohn's disease that it is not possible to say what the typical symptoms are. Most patients are likely to experience chest pain behind the breastbone, usually when they swallow.

Symptoms of Crohn's Disease of the Appendix

Appendicitis due to Crohn's disease may precede symptoms of Crohn's disease elsewhere in the gastrointestinal tract. However, Crohn's disease of the appendix can be present without symptoms in a patient who has symptoms of Crohn's disease elsewhere.

As with garden-variety appendicitis, the usual symptom is a sudden onset of pain low down on the right side of the abdomen.

Are People with Crohn's Disease Sick All the Time?

People with Crohn's disease are more likely than those with ulcerative colitis to experience persistent symptoms between flare-ups. But many patients are ill only intermittently. As with ulcerative colitis, attacks may occur every few weeks, months, or years. A person may have multiple flare-ups in one year and then none for several years, or any other irregular pattern that you can imagine. The average risk of a flare-up is about 30 percent per year.

Signs of Crohn's Disease

Unlike those with ulcerative colitis, many people with Crohn's have specific signs that, together with the symptoms, point quite strongly to the disease. About 25 percent of patients have an easily felt area of swelling, most commonly in the lower right part of the abdomen. This is much more distinct than the vague fullness that can be felt in some patients with ulcerative colitis. The swelling is often the size of a small grapefruit, and often as firm. The area is usually tender, and the tenderness can be anything from mild to extreme. If it is mild, the swelling is usually the result of inflamed intestine and surrounding tissues and enlarged lymph glands. If there is a marked tenderness, the swelling is usually due to a large abscess (boil). In this case the overlying skin may be red, and it may look stretched. In some patients, generally those with moderate tenderness, the swelling is due to a combination of swollen tissues and an abscess. In a thin patient, the swelling in the abdomen may be visible.

Another common sign of Crohn's disease is peri-anal disease (disease around the anus). This occurs in about 25 percent of patients and usually takes the form of a fistula (an abnormal connection between two organs), with or without one or more abscesses. Some patients have very swollen tags of skin around the anus. This finding is quite characteristic of Crohn's disease. Many healthy people who develop hemorrhoids get skin tags, but swelling of these tags is minimal.

FOUR

How Is IBD Diagnosed?

Physicians have an arsenal of tools to aid them in diagnosing inflammatory bowel disease.

Ulcerative Colitis

Ulcerative colitis is diagnosed from symptoms – frequent, urgent trips to the bathroom and bloody diarrhea – and the typically raw or scraped appearance of the rectum when the doctor examines it with an endoscope. During the examination of the rectum, the doctor will usually take a biopsy (tissue sample) to confirm the diagnosis. He or she may also arrange to have stools sent to a lab to check for infectious diseases that mimic ulcerative colitis.

Sigmoidoscopy

Usually a patient suspected of having ulcerative colitis will undergo a diagnostic procedure called sigmoidoscopy ("-oscopy" means to look into; to look into the sigmoid colon is "sigmoidoscopy"). It involves passing an instrument (a sigmoidoscope) through the anus into the rectum, and then into the sigmoid colon. The procedure allows the physician to view the mucosa (inner lining) of the bowel.

Colonoscopy

Colonoscopy (looking into the colon) is a diagnostic procedure in which the doctor examines most or all of the colon. It can be used to diagnose IBD and to determine how much of the colon is inflamed. During the procedure, the end of the ileum can also be examined in some people. Colonoscopy can be used, as well, to check for cancer (see Chapter 10). The procedure is usually done on an outpatient basis. Even if you have diarrhea, the colon needs to be cleaned out for colonoscopy Sedation is often given to relax you and minimize discomfort.

Preparation for Colonoscopy

The three most commonly used preparations for colonoscopy include electrolyte solutions, sodium phosphate solutions, and magnesium citrate. All can cause nausea, vomiting, abdominal fullness, and crampy abdominal pain. Occasionally, these side effects are so severe that the person is unable to continue taking the preparation. Through trial and error, most people find at least one preparation that they can tolerate. Additional information on two of these agents can be found in the sidebar in Chapter 6 dealing with constipation.

Air-contrast Barium Enema

Until colonoscopy became widely available, most people with ulcerative colitis had the extent of their disease estimated with an air-contrast barium enema, which is an X-ray of the colon. After the bowel has been appropriately cleansed, a short plastic tube is inserted into the rectum through the anus. Air and a suspension of barium sulfate (an inert substance easily visible on X-rays) are blown into the colon and multiple pictures are taken. Using a bit of barium and a lot of air, the radiologist (a physician specializing in interpreting X-rays) can usually coat the entire lining of the colon. The technique shows details of the inner lining of the colon, which is irregular instead of smooth in people with colitis.

Barium enemas are still commonly used. Family doctors who suspect ulcerative colitis may send you for one. A gastroenterologist or surgeon may also want you to undergo a barium enema. In some people it is not possible, for technical reasons, to pass the colonoscope all the way around the colon. In others, strictures (areas of narrowing) may prevent passage of the instrument.

Crohn's Disease

Crohn's disease is suspected when a person suffers abdominal cramps and diarrhea, with weight loss, for more than two weeks. A mass of swollen tissue that can be felt in the abdomen strongly increases the doctor's suspicion. Abscesses or fistulas around the anus are even stronger indicators.

Crohn's disease is diagnosed on the basis of X-rays more often than is ulcerative colitis. This is because most Crohn's disease is less accessible by colonoscope than is ulcerative colitis. Most Crohn's disease occurs in the ileum, or the ileum and the right side of the colon. It is neither practical nor possible to do a colonoscopy on every person suspected of having the disease. But someone with chronic diarrhea will very likely have a sigmoidoscopy as part of the investigation. Techniques for diagnosing Crohn's disease follow.

Single-Contrast Barium Enema

There are three ways to use X-rays to diagnose Crohn's disease in the ileum. The first is to do a single-contrast barium enema. The technique is the same as for an air-contrast barium enema, except that no air is used. Barium is run through the anus and rectum, then up the colon to the ileocecal valve (see Chapter 1) and into the end of the ileum, so it can be seen by X-ray.

Small-Bowel Series or Small-Bowel Follow-Through

The second method for examining the ileum with X-rays is to do a small-bowel series or a small-bowel follow-through (sometimes called a GI motor meal). You are given two or three large glasses of barium-sulfate suspension to drink. As the stomach empties the barium into the small intestine, X-rays are taken at set intervals until the barium arrives at the end of the ileum. At that time, the radiologist usually takes pictures of the end of the ileum. In most people with Crohn's of the ileum, the disease is obvious.

Small-Bowel Enema

The third technique for studying the ileum with X-rays is a small-bowel enema. A tube is passed through your nose, down the esophagus, through the stomach into the duodenum and then the jejunum (upper small bowel). Barium is injected through the tube by the radiologist and monitored as it progresses through the small bowel. The main advantage of this technique is that the pictures are sometimes more accurate than a small-bowel series. However, many people dislike the procedure intensely because of the tube. In the past few years, some radiologists have made the experience less uncomfortable by putting freezing in the nose before inserting the tube. Some also give intravenous medication to relax you.

Is Colonoscopy Used to Diagnose Crohn's Disease?

Abnormalities in the ileum can be missed with X-rays. In selected patients, colonoscopy is performed, passing the colonoscope all the way around the colon and into the ileum. Occasionally, Crohn's disease is diagnosed in this way even when an apparently normal ileum is clearly seen on X-rays. Some gastroenterologists prefer to *start* with colonoscopy in diagnosing

Crohn's disease, then proceed to X-rays later, if necessary. Crohn's disease of the colon can be diagnosed with sigmoidoscopy, colonoscopy, or barium enema.

Enteroscopy

Crohn's disease of the upper ileum or the jejunum is generally diagnosed by a small-bowel series or a small-bowel enema. On very rare occasions, a procedure known as enteroscopy is used to examine the jejunum or upper ileum directly. Your nose and throat are frozen with a spray, intravenous sedation is usually given, and a scope is passed down the esophagus, through the stomach, and into the small bowel to make or exclude a diagnosis of Crohn's disease.

Esophagogastroduodenoscopy

Crohn's disease of the esophagus, stomach, or duodenum is generally diagnosed by a procedure known as esophagogastroduodenoscopy. This involves passing a scope into the mouth and down the throat after appropriate freezing. Often referred to as OGD or EGD, the procedure is generally painless, or nearly so. Biopsies, which you don't feel, may be taken. Sedation is given to relax you if you are anxious about the procedure, and you may fall asleep, but this is *not* a general anesthetic.

Upper GI Series

Occasionally, Crohn's disease of the esophagus, stomach, or duodenum will be diagnosed with a barium X-ray known as an upper GI series. You drink a barium-sulfate suspension (generally flavored, which helps a little!), and a radiologist examines the esophagus, stomach, and duodenum and takes pictures.

Ultrasound

Within the past 15 years, it has become possible to use sound waves (ultrasound) to examine the bowel. Although this does not allow a specific diagnosis to be made, it can sometimes show a thickened bowel when someone is too ill to undergo routine diagnostic testing. Thickened bowel has several causes, but one of the more common ones is Crohn's disease. Ultrasound can also be used to diagnose certain complications of IBD, especially abscesses within the abdomen.

CAT (CT) Scan

In addition to diagnostic ultrasound, X-ray studies known as CAT scans (or CT scans) have proven useful in some cases. CAT stands for "computerized axial tomography." "Computerized" means the X-ray machine is controlled by a computer. "Tomography" refers to an X-ray technique whereby pictures of slices of your body are taken without slicing you up! "Axial" indicates that the X-rays are taken along the long axis of your body. A CAT scan of the abdomen starts with a slice across your body at the lower ribs and proceeds downward to your groin. CAT scans can show where the bowel is thick and, sometimes, where it is narrow. The main value of a CAT scan in IBD is that it shows the presence and location of the abscesses that occur as a complication of Crohn's disease (see Chapter 9).

Which Is Better – Ultrasound or a CAT Scan?

Ultrasound is believed to be perfectly safe. A CAT scan involves radiation. Generally speaking, ultrasound works better in thin people and CAT scans work better in overweight people. Fat has a distinctive appearance on a CAT scan and can outline various organs and structures. Gas in the bowel can greatly interfere with the transmission of sound waves, so if a patient has a bowel obstruction, or some other reason for having a lot of gas in the bowel, a CAT scan will be better.

Leukocyte (White Blood Cell) Scan

This test shows areas of intestinal inflammation by picking up concentrations of white blood cells. A small sample of your blood is removed and mixed with indium-111, a radioactive substance. The blood is injected back into you and a special camera, known as a gamma camera, moves back and forth over your abdomen, taking a kind of picture. The test is popular in some centers. However, it is not specific for Crohn's disease, and has no advantages over other methods of diagnosis in the vast majority of cases.

FIVE

Diet and IBD

Once the diagnosis of inflammatory bowel disease has been confirmed through tests, and other diseases have been ruled out, the question is how to treat it.

One of the areas of greatest interest to people with IBD is diet. They often experiment with changes in diet, sometimes even before they have received medical advice. People with Crohn's disease often discover that they feel better if they don't eat. Unfortunately this worsens the weight loss many patients experience. Some patients mistakenly believe that spicy or greasy food should be avoided, but then their diet becomes boring. This can lead to eating even less food and losing more weight.

When a patient is ill and needs drugs and/or surgery, sometimes maintaining adequate nutrition becomes an afterthought. But good nutrition is always desirable for those with IBD, as it is for everyone. Although anyone can call himself or herself a "nutritionist," in North America only registered dietitians, some doctors, some nurses, and some pharmacists are properly qualified to give accurate nutritional advice.

Most patients with IBD can eat a perfectly normal or near-normal diet most of the time. But when you are ill, sometimes avoiding certain foods is recommended, or a liquid diet is prescribed.

Lactose Intolerance

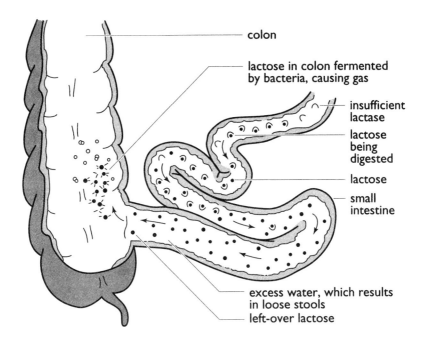

colon

lactose in colon fermented by bacteria, causing gas

insufficient lactase

lactose being digested

lactose

small intestine

excess water, which results in loose stools

left-over lactose

Common Dietary Restrictions in IBD

Lactose

Lactose is a sugar in dairy products, and is commonly known as "milk sugar." Some people with IBD have less pain, diarrhea, and gas if they restrict lactose in their diet.

In the inner lining of the small intestine, we all have a variety of enzymes (proteins that digest – "break down" – other chemicals). One of these enzymes is named "lactase," and its function is to digest lactose. When lactose is acted on by lactase, it is broken down into two simpler sugars: glucose and galactose. Both are rapidly and easily absorbed through the small intestine into the bloodstream.

As long as you have enough lactase enzyme for the lactose you take in, there is no problem. All the lactose will be digested, and the resulting glucose and galactose will be absorbed. But if you don't produce enough lactase, only some of the lactose will be digested. As the undigested lactose travels down the small intestine, it causes water to be drawn into the intestine by osmosis. This water is held in the intestine and may produce cramps. The extra fluid in the intestine may also cause loose bowel movements (diarrhea).

When this undigested lactose reaches the colon, it *is* digested, but by the bacteria we all have there. The process is known as fermentation. When lactose is fermented by bacteria, it is broken down into acids and lots of gas. The gas can cause a bloated feeling, pain in the abdomen, and an excess passage of gas from the rectum.

What Is Lactose Intolerance?

The symptoms – bloating, pain, diarrhea, gas – that result from a failure to digest lactose are referred to collectively as "lactose intolerance." Some people use the term "lactase deficiency." It really doesn't matter which term you use. The fact is that if you ingest more lactose than your small intestine can handle, you will have some or all of these symptoms.

Who Gets Lactose Intolerance?

As we get older we gradually lose some of our lactase enzyme, and thus are less able to process lactose-containing food. This doesn't happen to everyone, but it happens to many people. It is not serious; it is a nuisance. Of course it's unpleasant to have abdominal pain, diarrhea, or a lot of gas, but it's important to remember that it's not dangerous.

Lactose intolerance is more common in blacks and Asians than in Caucasians. As mentioned in Chapter 2, IBD is three times as common in Jews as in non-Jews. As it happens, lactose

---

Are You Lactose Intolerant?

Some doctors diagnose lactose intolerance by doing a lactose tolerance test. The most practical and direct way to determine lactose intolerance is to vary the amount of lactose in the diet.

Let's compare a couple of examples.

A 23-year-old woman developed ulcerative colitis. She was treated with medication but was also told to avoid all milk and milk products. Her disease came under good control. She was advised to stay on the low-lactose diet indefinitely. She consulted another gastroenterologist, because she was unhappy about having to avoid dairy products, and was told she should gradually increase her intake of milk and milk products. She was able to resume her usual habit of a glass of milk a day and cheese three to four times a week. There was no evidence of lactose intolerance.

A 38-year-old man was referred to a physician for a second opinion because he had persistent diarrhea with his Crohn's disease despite taking several medications. He said he had never tried any dietary restriction. He was in the habit of having cold cereal with milk every morning, cheese two or three times a week in a sandwich, yogurt occasionally, and ice cream frequently in the summer. He was advised to stop all milk, cheese, yogurt, and ice cream for one week, then report back. Prior to restricting his intake of lactose, he was having five to ten watery bowel movements a day with an excessive amount of gas. One week later he reported that he was having three to five bowel movements a day with much less gas. Because of this improvement, he was referred to a dietitian for advice on a strict lactose-free diet. Two weeks later, he was having one or two normal bowel movements a day. Clearly he was made completely better by eliminating lactose from his diet.

---

intolerance is also more common in Jews than in certain other ethnic groups. Lactose intolerance can occur in conjunction with IBD, but it is not the cause of IBD. It is also not an allergy. There is some evidence that lactose intolerance may be a little more common in patients with IBD than in other people, but this is not definite.

Patients who are not known to have lactose intolerance *may* experience it for the first time at the onset of their disease. It is worthwhile to avoid lactose to see if it makes a difference.

If it does not, then there is no point in avoiding it, because dairy products are a good source of nutrients and energy, and both are important when you are ill.

Remember that you cannot harm yourself by eating lactose-containing foods when you are ill with IBD, even if you have lactose intolerance. You may go to the bathroom more, you may have more abdominal discomfort, and you may have more gas, but this does not mean your disease has gotten worse. Obviously it may be difficult to tell what is going on if this happens, however, and the simple solution is to remove lactose from your diet temporarily.

Maintaining a Good Calcium Intake If You Are Lactose Intolerant
If you restrict the amount of lactose you take in, you may not get enough calcium, vitamin D, protein, and energy. There are ways to have dairy products but avoid the lactose they contain.

- Buy lactose-reduced milk. Pure lactase enzyme can be added to milk at the dairy. This enzyme predigests much of the lactose in the milk. Some people find that the milk tastes a little sweeter than normal milk, but few have any trouble getting used to it.

"Hidden" Lactose

Many foods contain lactose but may not be so labeled. An example is processed meat. Lactose is a cheap filler and is used liberally in hot dogs, for instance, to make them larger. Whey may be listed as an ingredient —it contains lactose, which may not be listed. Commercial gravies usually contain lactose because it can increase the volume of the gravy considerably. Interestingly, most breads are made with milk. One way to avoid them is to buy bread at a kosher Jewish bakery, where milk is not used in preparing bread. As well, many pills contain lactose. People with a marked lactose intolerance may experience symptoms if they take them.

Although people often talk about the "calories" in food, the scientifically correct term is "kilocalories" (there are 1,000 calories in a kilocalorie, or Kcal; the metric equivalent is 4.184 kilojoules). Because of this confusion, I prefer to use the term "energy" when I am discussing caloric intake in a general sense. Where specific Kcal values are given, they are the same as the so-called "calories" popularly referred to in dieting books and articles.

- Add lactase to milk yourself, and take lactase tablets just before and while eating foods containing lactose. Lactase enzyme is commercially available in both liquid and tablet form. The liquid form can be added to milk or yogurt, but needs 24 hours to reduce the lactose content. Tablets must be taken with the food. The tablets are especially handy when you are eating in a restaurant, as you may not know which foods contain dairy products or added lactose.
- Eat aged cheeses. Aging cheese reduces the amount of lactose in it because aging involves adding bacteria to cause fermentation. "Old" cheddar contains very little lactose and can be eaten comfortably by most people with lactose intolerance. Those with mild lactose intolerance can generally eat less aged cheeses, such as medium cheddar.
- Eat yogurt made with live/active bacterial culture. All yogurt is made with bacteria, but labeling identifies only those with live bacteria. The bacteria used produce lactase enzyme and release it. Thus at least some of the lactose in the yogurt can be digested.

Do You Need Extra Calcium If You Are Lactose Intolerant?
If you're trying a low-lactose diet, there is no urgency about

taking calcium pills. The body can easily do without the lost calcium for weeks, even months. In fact, many healthy adults have very little calcium in their diet, and in some people it doesn't make much difference. The body controls the blood calcium level the way a thermostat controls the temperature in a house. If the blood calcium level is a little low, then the body extracts calcium from the bones. Of course, this can make the bones soft and more prone to fracture. But other factors influence the strength of the bones, such as exercise, the amount of vitamin D in the diet, and exposure to sunlight, which leads to the formation of extra vitamin D in the skin.

Many adults develop osteoporosis as they get older. The use of glucocorticosteroids (often called steroids) such as prednisone to treat IBD increases the risk. It is well recognized that calcium can be added to the skeleton easily up to the age of 35. After 35 it becomes more difficult. However, providing enough calcium to prevent further deterioration seems to be effective.

Once you have established what level of lactose you can tolerate, having a registered dietitian assess the amount of calcium in your diet is useful.

Should You Take Calcium Pills?

If your calcium intake is below the recommended daily amount, you can decide whether to improve your intake, either by changing your diet or by taking calcium tablets. If you are going to take calcium tablets, tell your doctor. Calcium is absorbed more effectively in the presence of vitamin D. You can buy a calcium–vitamin D tablet. If you can't find a combined tablet that gives you the amount of calcium you need, you can buy calcium tablets alone and take the cheapest daily multivitamin pill to get the vitamin D you need. Remember that both vitamin D and calcium can be bad for you, as well as good for you. Too much of either one can make you seriously ill. Just because a little vitamin D is needed to help absorb calcium doesn't mean that a lot is better for you.

Some people get constipated on calcium and this may mean the dose has to be reduced. Taking excessive calcium can lead to kidney stones, and even calcium deposits in various organs and tissues, sometimes with serious results.

Numerous calcium tablets are available on the market. Some are "name brand"; those sold in large chain pharmacies are "house brand"; and there are others. Using calcium that comes from oyster shells has become popular. This is perfectly all right provided the product is reputable. Name-brand and house-brand tablets are generally acceptable. But you should know that oyster shells can be contaminated with undesirable elements such as arsenic.

Some people take bone-meal tablets. These are made from horse bones, some of which contain a lot of lead. Such tablets are *not* an advisable source of calcium.

What about "Roughage" or Fiber?

Fruit, vegetables, and grains are considered essential ingredients of a healthy, well-balanced diet.

Some of these foods have a laxative effect, and clearly this is undesirable when you are in the midst of a flare-up of IBD. These foods can also produce excessive gas, which may be particularly bothersome during a flare-up.

Two chemicals in fruit are likely to act as laxatives – sorbitol and fructose. Sorbitol is present primarily in prunes, peaches, pears, and apple juice. It is also used as a sweetener in many kinds of gum, in some mints, and in some liquid medications. We are unable to digest sorbitol, and have a limited ability to absorb fructose. We can handle some of either one without getting a laxative effect, but if an excess (which differs for different people) of one or both is taken in, then it acts just like lactose in a person with lactose intolerance. Like unabsorbed lactose, both cause water to be drawn into the intestine by osmosis and this leads to loose stools. And just like unabsorbed lactose, both are broken down in the colon by bacteria, releasing excessive gas.

Many vegetables and grains are a "natural" source of gas. The gas is produced when bacteria digest complex-carbohydrate residue in the colon. A relatively new enzyme product called Beano can predigest the fiber in these foods before it reaches the colon. The breakdown products do not include gas. Beano may be effective in reducing gas from peas and beans, nuts and seeds, grains and cereals, and a variety of vegetables. (A detailed list is available from the manufacturer.) Beano is used by mixing a few drops in with those foods that may produce gas. It is available in most pharmacies. People who are allergic to penicillin may also be allergic to Beano, because it is taken from a mold, just like penicillin.

A patient having a flare-up of IBD may well be more comfortable avoiding fruits and vegetables. Many patients can return to eating these foods between flare-ups. However, some people with IBD always have a degree of diarrhea and recognize that they are better off without these foods, good as they may be.

It is perfectly all right to experiment with different fruits and vegetables to see if you tolerate some better than others. Some patients know that they have to avoid foods that contain sorbitol but that they will have no difficulty with other fruit, such as berries.

People who have small-bowel Crohn's with a narrowing (stricture) in the small intestine may have particular difficulty with fibrous foods, because the stricture is fixed in size and cannot get wider, no matter how hard the intestine tries to push fibrous foods through. These patients may get crampy pain when they eat some fruits and vegetables.

Cereal fiber, such as bran, may not cause a problem for small-bowel Crohn's patients because bran can change shape and be squeezed through the narrowed areas. Bran may have to be avoided, though, because it is a potent laxative. It also produces troublesome gas in some cases.

Restricting fruits and vegetables necessarily means a decreased intake of minerals (potassium and iron) and vitamins (A, C, and folic acid). The solutions are to eat bananas (potassium); increase citrus juices, tomato juice, ketchup, and brown sugar (potassium, vitamin C); increase meat (iron and folic acid); increase milk and milk products (if you are not lactose intolerant) and liver (vitamin A); eat whole-grain cereals (fiber); and avoid only coarse fibers (celery, apple skins) and large seeds.

Fat

Some patients with small-bowel Crohn's disease do have to reduce the amount of fat in their diet, if the last three feet (about a meter) or more of the ileum is severely diseased, or has been surgically removed or bypassed (see Chapter 7). Fat absorption is very likely to be decreased and diarrhea will result or, if already present, will likely be aggravated. This results in a loss of energy intake (and probably a loss of weight).

How Can a Patient on a Low-Fat Diet Compensate?
If you are on a low-fat diet, can maintain an acceptable weight, and are not bothered by the fat restriction, there is nothing you need do. But if you need to gain weight, or you would like to use fat for salad dressing or cooking, there is a manufactured

food product you can use. It is known as MCT, which stands for "medium-chain triglyceride." A considerable number of nutritional products contain MCTs, but there are only two products in which MCTs make up all or most of the fat.

The first is *MCT oil*. This is a pure liquid oil product derived from coconut oil. Many people take it as they would any liquid medication. It can also be mixed with fruit juices, used on salads and other vegetables, incorporated into sauces, or used in other cooking and baking. The second product comes as a powder and must be mixed with water prior to use.

Individuals with advanced cirrhosis of the liver must use these products with caution because large amounts can cause drowsiness or confusion.

Clear Fluid Diets

Sometimes it is necessary to avoid all food except for clear fluids. In certain situations this can improve your symptoms dramatically – particularly if you have small-bowel Crohn's disease and especially if the symptoms are due to a partial small-bowel obstruction.

If you are in hospital and have not been allowed to eat or drink *anything*, clear fluids are wonderful, even enjoyable for a day or two. After that, this diet gets pretty boring, not to mention that it is very poor nutritionally. It supplies only 400 to 600 kilocalories (1,700 to 2,500 kilojoules) per day, with

A Typical Clear Fluid Diet

Breakfast	Lunch	Dinner
jelly	jelly	jelly
apple juice	apple juice	apple juice
tea with sugar	chicken broth	beef broth
	tea with sugar	tea with sugar

about 135 grams of carbohydrate, 8 grams of protein, and no fat. A person weighing 150 pounds (about 70 kilos) needs at least 1,500 kilocalories (6,300 kilojoules), 60 grams of protein, and a small amount of fat each day. So it is important for both you and your doctor to remember that you should not be on clear fluids for more than a few days.

Full Fluid Diets

A patient doing well on a clear fluid diet may move to a full fluid diet. A typical full fluid diet provides 1,100 to 1,300 kilocalories (4,600 to 5,400 kilojoules) a day, and usually contains at least 165 grams of carbohydrate, 40 grams of protein, and an equivalent amount of fat. If lactose intolerance is not a problem, this diet is certainly a great improvement over a clear fluid diet, though it does not include enough energy or protein for most patients recovering from an illness or an operation. If you are lactose intolerant, a full fluid diet cannot be used, since many of the foods in it contain dairy products. In fact, if you subtract the dairy products from the full fluid diet, you are pretty well back to clear fluids. Furthermore, a lot of older people don't like sugar and don't like milk products. This is important to remember, because older people are more vulnerable to various illnesses and complications, especially if they are malnourished.

A Typical Full Fluid Diet

Breakfast	Lunch	Dinner
orange juice	blended juice	pineapple juice
strained oatmeal	strained cream soup	strained cream soup
2% milk	custard	ice cream
brown sugar	2% milk	2% milk
coffee or tea with	coffee or tea with	coffee or tea with
sugar and cream	sugar and cream	sugar and cream

Why Restrict All Solids?

The purpose of restricting solids is to eliminate most residue (indigestible matter). This is important for patients with small-bowel Crohn's disease with partial obstruction or an acute flare-up, but also for patients with fistulas (due to Crohn's disease or as a complication of surgery) or people with short-bowel syndrome (see TPN, below). But as we've seen, restricting solids in the diet results in an inadequate intake of energy and some nutrients.

Elemental Diets, Polymeric Diets, and Modular Products

In the past 25 years a wide range of specialized nutritional products has been developed to insure adequate nutrition for patients on fluids.

An "elemental diet" is one in which all nutrients are in their simplest forms. The carbohydrate is present as glucose; the protein is present as amino acids; any fat that is present (usually very little) is in the form of long-chain or medium-chain triglycerides. These components are mixed with all the necessary vitamins, minerals, and trace elements. In concept, the elemental diet is "predigested." In reality, however, the fat supplied requires some digestion. These products are generally available in a powdered form and must be dissolved in water and used within 48 hours.

"Polymeric diets" contain complex chemical forms of the various nutrients. For example, carbohydrate might be present in the form of corn syrup; protein is often in the form of casein (this is milk protein – it has nothing to do with lactose); and fat may be in the form of corn oil. Natural chemicals such as carrageenan or other ingredients may be added to make these diets more palatable. Most of these products are marketed in liquid form in cans or boxes. A few of the polymeric diets are very low in fat. Some come in powdered form and must be mixed with water before use. The canned or boxed products generally have a shelf life of approximately two years. However, once a can or a box has been opened it must be refrigerated and completely used within 48 hours. The majority of these products are lactose-free.

"Modular products" supply one particular nutrient. The medium-chain triglyceride product to replace fat is an example of a modular product.

When Are Liquid Diets Used in IBD?

- *Ulcerative colitis:* There are times when a patient with ulcerative colitis does not feel like eating much but is willing to drink. Since most ordinary fluids are filling without supplying a lot of energy, liquid diet products can prove very useful. It is also possible to have high-energy, nutritious liquids that are not manufactured. The two best examples are milkshakes and eggnog; they are high in both energy and protein. However, because they also contain a lot of lactose, some patients with lactose intolerance cannot use them. If a patient with ulcerative colitis can eat a reasonably normal diet, there is no advantage to using specialized products. Nutritional therapy alone is not a treatment for ulcerative colitis.
- *Crohn's disease:* Unlike ulcerative colitis, nutritional therapy alone is an effective treatment for Crohn's disease, especially when the disease is active in the small bowel. In adults, these diets are most often used by patients who want to avoid using steroids to treat the problem, by doctors who want their patients to avoid steroids, or by patients who want to stop using steroids but have been unable to do so. Most patients who go on a liquid diet will be able to reduce steroids without

---

About Steroids

The term "steroids" is commonly used to refer to a large number of hormones that have similar chemical structure. They include glucocorticoid steroids (which can reduce inflammation), male sex hormones (such as the so-called anabolic steroids sometimes misused by athletes), female sex hormones, and others.

In this book the term "steroids" refers exclusively to glucocorticoid steroids.

---

having a flare-up. A substantial number will be able either to stay off steroids or to use a reduced dose when the liquid-diet course is finished and a regular diet has been resumed. Although it was initially thought that the diet had to be elemental, it has been conclusively shown that polymeric diets are just as good. There is still some controversy about whether all polymeric diets are equal. Liquid-diet therapy is almost as effective as prednisone, the steroid most commonly used for Crohn's disease.

How Do Liquid-Diet Products Work?
So far, we don't know exactly why this type of therapy works. Since these products are sterilized and most regular food is not, many researchers have thought that certain components of bacteria aggravate the inflammation of Crohn's disease. There is also some evidence that simply making sure you eat properly can have a beneficial effect on Crohn's disease.

Does Liquid-Diet Therapy Work for Everyone?
No treatment for Crohn's disease works for all patients, and this is no exception. This type of therapy works particularly well in patients with small-bowel Crohn's disease, but not in all such patients. It works much less often in patients with Crohn's disease of the colon.

Tube Feeding

There are three situations in which liquid diets are taken by tube. They are:

1. when a patient cannot drink enough to achieve an energy goal because he or she cannot find a product that is palatable;
2. to reduce or prevent side effects such as nausea or diarrhea;
3. to administer a product which is meant to be given by tube, usually because it is simply undrinkable because of its taste or some other feature.

The tube is inserted into the stomach through the nose. This sounds unpleasant, but the tubes are small and soft, and generally they are well tolerated. Although the liquid diet can be dripped in through the tube using gravity alone, it is often administered using a pump. For some patients, controlling the rate of delivery with the pump is important; for others it is not. Battery-operated pumps allow patients to move around both in and out of hospital.

Some adults will do almost anything to avoid being tube-fed. Children, on the other hand, adapt well to this form of treatment (see Chapter 8).

Advantages of Liquid-Diet Therapy

If nutritional therapy is to be used, one of the greatest advantages of a liquid diet is that it can be done on an outpatient basis in the majority of cases.

It is also a safe means of treatment, provided the doctor or dietitian instructing you is familiar with it. Patients on this type of diet do not have to stay home. They can go to work, school, or anywhere else. As long as they are able to consume the desired amount of energy per day, they really have no restrictions whatsoever on their activities.

Disadvantages of Liquid-Diet Therapy

Nevertheless, liquid-diet therapy has several disadvantages. One is cost. Of course, when you are not eating a regular diet, that cost saving must be taken into account. But generally it does not cancel out the cost of the specialized diet. Unfortunately, insurance companies rarely pay for these products, claiming they are "food" and not "treatment." Some government health plans do pay, but for specific groups only.

A second disadvantage is taste fatigue. Many people find they can take these products for a few days but get bored with the taste after that. Even when patients can handle these products for longer, most prefer one flavor. This again leads to taste fatigue. Using a variety of clear fluids, flavorings, or recipes helps. Water-based products, for example, can be made into a slush or even frozen like "Popsicles."

Ultimately you will have to stop the liquid-diet therapy. Even if you feel perfectly well on a liquid diet, only after you stop the diet will you and the doctor know if anything has really been accomplished. As soon as you go back on regular food, your previous symptoms of Crohn's disease may immediately reappear.

Additional problems for some patients on liquid diets include nausea, a perpetual feeling of unpleasant fullness, abdominal cramps, and frequent or loose stools. Obviously some of these side effects can easily be confused with the Crohn's disease that is being treated. Although some patients have one small bowel movement every few days, one to three loose movements a day should not be considered a problem.

Can You Have Any Regular Food While on a Liquid Diet?

Many of these products do not provide enough water. I tell

my patients to take the liquid diet when hungry and clear fluids when thirsty. They can also have clear fluids to combat taste fatigue, provided that they still achieve their daily energy goal.

How Long Should You Stay on a Liquid Diet?

There are no rules about how long to stay on a liquid diet and a lot depends on your physician's experience. I tell my patients that they have to fulfill two conditions before they can go back to regular food. First, they have to take the liquid diet for a minimum of two weeks. Second, they must feel perfectly well for a minimum of one week. If a patient feels much better but not perfectly well and has not improved further for a week, then I compromise and accept partial improvement. Generally, the maximum period I prescribe a liquid diet for is eight weeks.

TPN – Total Parenteral Nutrition

In the term "total parenteral nutrition" or TPN, "total" refers to providing a nutritionally complete diet; "parenteral" means that the diet is given by a route other than the GI tract. In the late 1960s, it became possible to feed people high-energy diets intravenously. (North American researchers were instrumental in pioneering this technology.) This meant that people with Crohn's disease could avoid food, improve, and still receive adequate nutrition.

In the 1970s this was a popular treatment for the disease. However, in the late 1970s and through the early 1980s it became increasingly obvious that most such people could be equally well treated with oral liquid diets. As awareness of the risks and expense of TPN grew, more and more patients were treated with liquid diets, frequently on an outpatient basis. For some, nutritional therapy was a combination of a liquid diet and parenteral nutrition (PN).

Today, TPN or supplemental PN is reserved mainly for patients who are acutely ill, such as those with severe colitis or toxic megacolon (see Chapter 9). Many of these patients can't or won't eat enough to maintain adequate nutrition. Occasionally some patients with Crohn's disease need prolonged temporary or even permanent PN to maintain adequate nutrition. Others require a long period of nutritional build-up prior to surgery and cannot take in food through the GI tract. Still others – fortunately not very many – have had most of their small bowel removed surgically and don't have enough intestine left to absorb all nutrients (short-bowel syndrome). Such patients receive HPN, or home parenteral nutrition. Just as with home tube feeding, patients on HPN become quite knowledgeable and self-reliant about administering the intravenous (IV) diet and maintaining the IV site. Some hospitals have HPN programs to teach the technique.

The main advantages of TPN at the present time are that it can prevent or reduce nutritional deterioration in seriously ill patients, and it can be a virtual lifeline to patients unable to get proper nutrition because of an inadequate amount of intestine.

The main disadvantages are that TPN is highly specialized and expensive. Furthermore, the need to have foreign material (the IV line) in the body constantly puts the patient at risk of blood infections and blood clots – both potentially life-threatening complications.

High-Glutamine Products
Glutamine is a nonessential amino acid. "Nonessential" means that the body is able to produce it, in comparison with "essential" amino acids, which must be taken in because the body is unable to manufacture them.

During physical stresses such as surgery or severe illness, the body may need more glutamine than it can produce.

Recent research has demonstrated that glutamine is an important nutrient for the jejunum. This has led some manufacturers of nutritional support products to promote high-glutamine products. But there is little evidence that glutamine is beneficial to the ileum, where the majority of small-bowel Crohn's disease occurs, and there is no conclusive evidence that high-glutamine products offer any special benefit to patients with Crohn's disease generally.

Some Unnecessary Dietary Restrictions in IBD

Some patients need to restrict their diet all the time, others need to do it some of the time, and some patients can always eat a perfectly normal diet.

Many patients, however, restrict their diets unnecessarily. Sometimes the doctor has imposed these restrictions, but in other cases they are self-imposed.

For example, many people avoid foods they can recognize in their bowel movements because of the mistaken belief that there is something wrong with their digestion. Humans cannot digest (break down) many of the components of dietary fiber. If you eat corn, you will see corn in your stool. The same is true for a large variety of skins, seeds, and other fibrous foods. This is normal.

Is It Necessary to Avoid Fried or Spicy Foods?

For the vast majority of IBD patients, there is absolutely no need to avoid fried or spicy foods. Many patients with IBD are underweight, particularly when they have been ill, and fat is an excellent source of energy. Fried foods not only taste good, but help you regain lost weight. Spices improve taste, which helps to increase food intake.

I am not suggesting you eat a high-fat diet, since fat may increase the risk of heart disease and other diseases in some people. But when you're trying to regain weight, it is generally harmless to eat an increased amount of fat. When I have a patient who is having trouble gaining weight after a flare-up of IBD, I often suggest high-fat, high-energy foods such as bacon and eggs, potato chips, and various fried foods.

Adverse Effects of Unnecessary Restrictions

If you avoid two or three foods because you think they may increase your symptoms, it's generally not a problem. But if you have a long list of foods that you avoid, it's likely that your disease is active and needs specific therapy. Avoiding a large number of foods usually decreases your appetite, because your diet becomes boring. Eating less, of course, reduces the amount of energy you take in, which leads to weight loss. A patient with active disease is likely already underweight, and losing more weight is undesirable.

Three Steps to Avoiding Self-imposed Dietary Restrictions

1. Avoid restrictions based on hearsay. When I ask patients why they are avoiding certain foods, they sometimes tell me that they "heard somewhere" that such a food "could" cause symptoms. Friends are rarely a reliable source of medical or nutritional advice. Relatives can be even worse, because they *care* about you.
2. If you think you've found a relationship between certain foods and certain symptoms, discuss your theory with your physician before you limit yourself permanently.
3. If you're older, especially if you live alone, put more effort into preparing meals. Otherwise your diet will be boring,

you'll eat less, and you'll lose weight. Older people, especially when they are ill, need balanced meals.

Remember, dietary restrictions should be discussed with your doctor or a registered dietitian. You can experiment yourself, but do not maintain any long-term restrictions without letting your doctor know.

S I X

Drugs and IBD

Before getting into the details of drug therapy, I must remind you of the old saying "A little learning is a dangerous thing." Knowledge is good, but it must be in context. Some people see the side effects of medications (or other treatments) and say, "Wow, look at the risks! I'm not going to do that!" But *not* doing something may also have risks. Not taking the treatment may mean that the illness will get worse or more complicated. The potential benefits and risks of any decision should be carefully considered by you and your doctor.

It's also important to be aware that there are "generic" side effects that have nothing to do with particular medications. For example, many tablets contain lactose, and some people have such extreme lactose intolerance (see Chapter 5) that this will affect them. Some tablets are large and difficult to swallow. A variety of medications used in IBD are taken in the form of an enema; there is a small but real risk of puncturing the rectum with the plastic enema tip.

Drugs used to treat IBD can be divided into two categories. The first includes those that reduce inflammation; this in turn reduces symptoms such as diarrhea and pain. The second includes those that have no effect on inflammation but may be useful in reducing or eliminating symptoms, especially diarrhea and crampy pain. In both categories, not all side effects are discussed, due to space limitations. There are also several nondrug therapies, such as dietary changes, covered in Chapter 5, and surgery, which we'll cover in Chapter 7.

Drugs That Reduce Inflammation

Sulfasalazine

In the late 1930s, Dr. Nana Svartz, a Swedish researcher, proposed linking one of the newly discovered sulfa drugs with acetylsalicylic acid (ASA, also called aspirin in the U.S.) to treat the painful joint disease rheumatoid arthritis, at that time thought to be caused by an infection. The first patient Dr. Svartz treated with such a combined drug, called sulfasalazine, happened to have ulcerative colitis as well. The most striking benefit for this patient was control of his colitis. Until the introduction of sulfasalazine in 1942, no medication had been able to control colitis. For the next eight years it remained the *only* drug available for the treatment of colitis, until 1950, when cortisone was introduced. Sulfasalazine continued to be the only drug in its class until the 1980s, when pure 5-ASA (5-aminosalicylate, the active ingredient of sulfasalazine) became available.

Many gastroenterologists now prefer to prescribe the newer 5-ASA drugs, but some still start with sulfasalazine. It's just as effective, it's cheaper, and it's familiar. The only drawback compared with pure 5-ASA is that sulfasalazine more often has side effects.

How Does It Work?

The 5-aminosalicylate (5-ASA) portion of the sulfasalazine, the active ingredient, limits the production of certain chemical products of inflammation that promote diarrhea. It also removes oxygen radicals from tissues. These substances, released during inflammation, are toxic to cells. Like all sulfa drugs, sulfasalazine is an antibacterial agent. This means that it prevents some bacteria from functioning and causing illness, although it does not kill them. At the present time, the antibacterial activity is not thought to be important in ulcerative colitis. It may have some value in Crohn's disease, but there is not much evidence for this, even though antibiotics – which *kill* bacteria – are clearly beneficial.

When Is It Used?
Sulfasalazine can be used to treat mild to moderate attacks of ulcerative colitis and Crohn's disease. But it is most valuable because it markedly *reduces the chance* of a flare-up of ulcerative colitis in most patients. If taken regularly, it continues to have this effect indefinitely. This does not guarantee you will not have a flare-up, but for most patients it significantly lessens the risk. A similar effect has not been proven in Crohn's disease, but some patients appear to do well on the drug. Sulfasalazine has not been shown to reduce the risk of Crohn's disease coming back after surgery. It is also used to treat arthritis, which occurs in about 20 percent of people with IBD.

What Are the Side Effects?
The most frequent side effects of sulfasalazine are gastrointestinal. Nausea and reduced appetite are common, but of course these can also be symptoms of IBD. Vomiting is less common. These side effects can sometimes be prevented if you start with a small dose of the drug and build it up slowly, rather than starting with a full dose on the first day. It also helps to take the pills with food and not on an empty stomach. A coated form of sulfasalazine releases the drug more slowly,

and is particularly helpful in reducing any nausea due to the drug.

The second most common type of side effect is an allergic reaction. This usually appears as an itchy rash (hives) or swelling of the hands and/or some or all of the face. In someone who has never taken the drug before, the reaction generally occurs 14 to 21 days after starting the drug. In someone who has taken the drug before, it generally occurs within the first week. Report any allergic reactions to your doctor immediately. About 70 percent of the people who have an allergic reaction to this drug can be desensitized, so that the drug can be gradually reintroduced. Occasionally allergic reactions will be associated with arthritis (inflamed joints), hepatitis (inflamed liver), fever, or many other inflammations of tissues and organs.

The third type of common side effect involves the blood. Red blood cells normally have a life span of 120 days. These blood cells are then taken up by the spleen, destroyed, and replaced by new red blood cells from the bone marrow, in a normal process that goes on all the time. In some patients, sulfasalazine causes the red blood cells to be destroyed prematurely. This process is called hemolysis, from "heme," meaning blood, and "lysis," meaning breakdown. Hemolysis is generally reversible and can be controlled in some patients simply by reducing the dose of sulfasalazine; in others, the drug must be stopped completely.

Folic acid (also known as folate) is one of the B vitamins, and one of the building blocks of red blood cells. Another blood-related side effect of sulfasalazine is that it can reduce the ability of the intestine to absorb folic acid, possibly leading to anemia. Physicians will prescribe a daily folic acid pill when necessary.

A rare but serious side effect of sulfasalazine is bone-marrow shutdown (marrow aplasia). In addition to red blood cells, the bone marrow makes white blood cells and platelets. With this side effect, the production of any or all types of blood cells may stop. Treatments for this exist but are not always effective, and death can result. Bone-marrow shutdown usually occurs within the first three months of therapy, but it also represents the most serious long-term risk of sulfasalazine. Unusual bleeding or bruising should be reported immediately to your doctor. Occasionally sulfasalazine can reduce a man's sperm count enough to make him infertile. Stopping the drug allows the count to return to normal, though this may take up to three months. Headaches can also occur with sulfasalazine. In some people they are mild, but in others they are severe enough that the drug must be stopped. Many patients who take sulfasalazine notice that their urine is orange-yellow. Yellowing of the skin and soft contact lenses has occasionally been reported, but this discoloration is harmless.

Sulfasalazine comes in tablets, either coated or uncoated; in a liquid form (suspension) that is orange-lemon in flavor and odor; or as an enema. A suppository form of the drug has been available in Europe for many years, but it has never been on the market in North America.

5-Aminosalicylate (5-ASA)
The active ingredient in sulfasalazine, 5-ASA, does not have any antibacterial properties. Although it is chemically similar to ASA, 5-ASA doesn't do anything that ASA does, and ASA doesn't do anything that 5-ASA does. This drug was introduced in North America in the 1980s and is now widely used.

How Does It Work?
Like sulfasalazine, 5-ASA reduces the production of certain

Because brands of drugs come and go, I have used generic ("no-name") drug names. For the brand names available in late 1996, see the drug table at the end of the book.

chemicals in the intestine that cause diarrhea. It also inactivates oxygen radicals that destroy tissue.

When Is It Used?

5-ASA can be used to treat mild to moderate attacks of ulcerative colitis and Crohn's disease. For people with proctitis or colitis limited to the last one to two feet (30 to 60 centimeters) of the colon, small doses taken rectally are frequently more effective than much larger doses taken orally. The drug is also used to reduce the chance of flare-ups of both these diseases in many patients. Used postoperatively, 5-ASA has been shown to reduce the risk of recurrent small-bowel Crohn's disease.

What Are the Side Effects?

Many of the side effects of 5-ASA are similar to those of sulfasalazine. But they occur much less commonly, because the sulfa portion of sulfasalazine responsible for many of those adverse effects is absent in 5-ASA.

Common side effects include nausea, headaches, and diarrhea. The diarrhea occurs more with some forms of the drug than with others. It can be reduced by introducing the drug gradually and taking the pills with food.

Other less common side effects include allergic reactions (e.g., itchy rash and swelling of the hands and face, and/or fever). As with sulfasalazine, some allergic patients can be desensitized. A severe, dull, steady pain across the upper abdomen may indicate pancreatitis (inflammation of the pancreas). If pancreatitis occurs, 5-ASA cannot be used again.

In rare cases, an attack of ulcerative colitis, or a worsening of an attack, will occur with 5-ASA. The drug must be stopped and the attack treated in some other way.

Hair loss has occasionally been reported as a side effect, but the reliability of the reports is questionable. There is a normal process of hair turnover, in which a certain number of hairs fall out every day and are replaced by new ones. It is extremely common for this turnover to be accelerated during an illness, and especially in the weeks afterwards. You may notice more hair in your comb or brush, and more hair in the shower or bathtub. If you have long hair, you are much more likely to be aware of this. But the loss is temporary; new hair is growing in. Hair loss is serious only if the hair comes out in clumps and leaves bald patches. To the best of my knowledge, this latter type of hair loss is extremely rare with 5-ASA.

Patients commonly use 5-ASA enemas or suppositories as maintenance therapy. The chronic use of any sort of enema or suppository can irritate the anal canal and produce pain and bleeding.

Research has suggested that kidney damage *may* be a side effect of long-term use of this drug. It is not unusual for patients on 5-ASA to have an excessive number of white blood cells in the urine. Having your urine and kidney function checked periodically when you use 5-ASA long-term is recommended until we know more about the importance of this effect.

5-ASA is available in tablets, enemas, and suppositories. A rectal foam has been used in clinical studies in Europe but is not currently available in North America.

There are several brands of 5-ASA tablets available at the present time. Each brand "targets" the 5-ASA to specific sites in the intestine. Whether these differences are of clinical significance has not yet been demonstrated. In addition to 5-ASA, other generic names for these products include mesalamine, mesalazine, and olsalazine.

Common Questions about 5-ASA

Q: Is one 5-ASA product better than any other for the treatment of small-bowel Crohn's disease?

A: The 5-ASA products that target the small bowel and colon are all approximately equal; the minor differences in formulation have not been studied comparatively.

Q: Is there any evidence that a person with colitis should be treated with a 5-ASA product that is targeted specifically at the colon?

A: While there are some published data suggesting that this is the case, the evidence is not compelling. It appears that all the oral forms are effective in colitis.

Q: Is there any point in trying 5-ASA enemas or suppositories if oral 5-ASA does not appear to be working?

A: Definitely yes! Rectally administered 5-ASA is often effective (even in very small doses) when oral 5-ASA is not (even in maximum doses).

Q: If I am doing well on sulfasalazine, should I switch to a "pure" 5-ASA product?

A: Most gastroenterologists agree that you should not "rock the boat." There is a somewhat greater risk of diarrhea as a side effect with 5-ASA; this is unpredictable and occasionally severe.

Q: If my ulcerative colitis has been inactive for several years, should I stop my sulfasalazine or 5-ASA medication?

A: Not without asking your doctor. The main function of these medications is to reduce the risk of a flare-up.

Steroids

The steroids used in IBD, known as glucocorticosteroids or glucocorticoids, are derivatives of cortisol, a natural steroid produced by the adrenal glands, which sit on top of the kidneys. Glucocorticoids are different from the anabolic steroids used by some athletes to enhance performance, and also used by doctors to treat certain diseases. The first glucocorticoid to be given to patients was cortisone, in 1950. The introduction of this potent drug revolutionized the treatment of many chronic diseases, including IBD. Currently the most-used glucocorticoid is prednisone.

How Do These Steroids Work?
Quite simply, glucocorticoids reduce inflammation.

When Are They Used?
These drugs are used to treat most moderate and severe attacks of ulcerative colitis and Crohn's disease. In patients with ulcerative colitis, once the attack has settled down significantly, the dose should gradually be reduced to zero over several weeks. In most patients with ulcerative colitis, there is no evidence that steroids prevent flare-ups of the disease, so patients should generally not remain on this medication between attacks. About 5 percent of patients with ulcerative colitis have what is referred to as "chronic continuous colitis." With these patients it may not be possible to get the dosage down to zero between attacks. Many of them require continuous steroid therapy to stay well.

It is much more common for patients to require continuous steroid therapy in Crohn's disease, to suppress chronic symptoms not controllable by other measures. However, many patients with Crohn's disease require steroids only intermittently. Still others do not need them at all. Steroids do not prevent Crohn's disease from recurring after surgery.

When either form of colitis is limited to the last one to two feet (30 to 60 centimeters) of the colon, glucocorticoids may be just as effective rectally as similar or larger doses taken orally, with fewer side effects.

What Are the Side Effects?
Steroids have both visible and invisible side effects.

Visible side effects: The visible side effects are more upsetting to you than to your doctor. It's not that your doctor doesn't care, but he or she knows that these effects are reversible weeks to months after the drug has been stopped. Also, these side effects are not dangerous in themselves. They include:

- rounding of the face – appears gradually;
- redness of the face, usually mild – creates a "healthier" appearance;
- increased appetite and weight gain, usually desirable;
- mood changes – often happier because of feeling better; feeling nervous or jittery; serious extremes of mood such as euphoria or severe depression are very uncommon;
- acne – mild to severe; may require antibiotics; mostly in individuals taking steroids for weeks or more; usually improves with dose reduction, but occasionally first appears, or becomes much worse, shortly after steroids stopped;
- increased energy and insomnia – some people sleep fewer hours than usual and yet do not get sleepy during the day;
- ankle swelling, in malnourished people;
- weakness of the muscles of the thighs and upper arms – difficulty climbing stairs and getting up from a seat without using your arms;
- night sweats – may also be a sign of illness;
- facial hair growth – rarely noticeable;
- skinny arms and a pot belly – with long-term therapy (years);
- a hump of fat on the middle of the upper back – with long-term therapy (years);
- thinning of the skin and easy bruising; mainly with long-term therapy;
- reduced growth rate and delayed puberty;

- muscle and joint stiffness soon after a course of oral steroids is completed.

Invisible side effects: These are of greater concern to your doctor, because they can cause irreversible harm. They include:

- softening of the bones – especially hips and spine; mainly with long-term therapy (years) but occasionally with short-term (weeks); physical inactivity, malnutrition, and a low-lactose diet increase risk, which can now be monitored with bone densitometry;
- reduced immunity – increased risk of infections; mainly with high doses and hospitalized patients;
- aggravation of diabetes mellitus– increased blood sugar, usually temporary;
- cataracts – mainly with higher doses and prolonged therapy;
- increased eye pressure (glaucoma) – more common in children;
- reduced potassium level, also a result of diarrhea; can contribute to weakness;
- high blood pressure – very uncommon;
- ulcers of the stomach and/or duodenum (controversial); only with high doses, if at all.

Stopping Steroids
The last invisible side effect may occur days to months after you stop taking steroids. Your body normally makes cortisol in the adrenal glands. When it is subjected to physical stress (e.g., fever, surgery, etc.), it produces up to ten times more cortisol. With *extreme* psychological stress, there can be a very temporary increase in cortisol. When you take a

Important Points to Remember about Glucocorticoid Steroid Therapy

- Never stop steroids suddenly, unless clearly advised to do so by your doctor. The usual practice is to taper the dose until it is down to zero, although if steroids have been taken for two weeks or less they can be stopped abruptly, if this is desired.
- Always advise any physician, dentist, or paramedical person treating you that you are or have been on steroids within the previous 12 months. Some physicians recommend that you wear a medical-alert bracelet if you're on steroids.
- Remind your own physician that you have been on steroids within the previous 12 months if you are being treated for an acute illness. Your doctor must keep track of hundreds of patients; you have only one — you!

glucocorticoid, normal cortisol production decreases or stops completely. When you stop taking the steroid, production begins again, but may be sluggish for up to a year. This means that you may need extra steroids at a time of physical stress, for up to 12 months after you have come off the medication. The extra steroids may be necessary for days or longer, depending on the illness. If the stress is mental, the dose should be increased only for one to two days, *if at all*. Symptoms of insufficient cortisol are nonspecific. They include nausea, extreme fatigue, weakness, light-headedness, and possibly diarrhea. If you suspect that you are not producing enough cortisol soon after stopping steroids, *discuss it with your doctor*.

Forms of Steroids

There are many different forms of cortisonelike steroids. They are available as pills (e.g., prednisone), suppositories (e.g., hydrocortisone), enemas (hydrocortisone, betamethasone, budesonide, tixocortol), rectal foams (hydrocortisone), and injectable forms (e.g., hydrocortisone, methylprednisolone, ACTH).

Newer steroids include tixocortol and budesonide enemas, on the market in Canada but not the U.S., and budesonide capsules, approved for Canada as of 1997 but not yet for the U.S. Others, such as fluticasone and prednisone metasulfabenzoate, are being studied in Europe. These drugs have fewer side effects because they act locally at the site of disease in the intestine and are absorbed into the bloodstream less, and/or are metabolized (broken down) more rapidly into inactive components.

Other Points about Steroids
If you need long-term steroid therapy, your doctor may tell you to try taking a double dose every second day and skipping the days in between – so-called alternate-day dosing. It is supposed to be just as effective, with fewer net side effects. However, many people complain that they simply do not feel as well on the "off" days, so this is not widely used.

People being treated with rectal steroids can often retain suppositories or foam much more easily than liquid enemas, sometimes with equal benefit.

Immunosuppressive Drugs
Immunosuppressives are another class of drugs used in the treatment of IBD. They were originally introduced to treat certain cancers. They have also been used to help prevent rejection in organ transplants. In both these situations, relatively large doses of the drugs are administered. It has been known for more than 30 years, however, that much smaller doses can be used effectively to treat a variety of other conditions, including IBD.

How Do They Work?
Immunosuppressive drugs reduce inflammation. How they do

this is not known. Since the immune system is thought to be overactive in IBD, their ability to suppress it may be important.

When Are They Used?

These drugs are most often used when there is a desire to reduce, eliminate, or avoid the use of steroids. Both ulcerative colitis patients and Crohn's disease patients who need frequent or continuous steroid therapy can often reduce their dosage, or even stop steroids altogether, if they take these drugs.

Immunosuppressives are generally considered only after agents such as sulfasalazine, 5-ASA, and antibiotics (Crohn's disease only) have proven unsatisfactory.

In ulcerative colitis, immunosuppressive drugs usually work within about 12 weeks, if there is going to be a response. Because some of these drugs act so slowly in Crohn's disease, you may have to wait up to 6 months or more, though some people respond more quickly. Because the drugs act so slowly, it is often necessary to increase steroids temporarily.

Here is a typical case. A 27-year-old man with Crohn's disease sought a second opinion because he could not stop taking steroids. He had a history of extensive surgery, so another operation was undesirable. Despite steroids, he was having daily crampy pain and diarrhea. He was put on 6-mercaptopurine (6-MP). One month later, he was told to try to reduce the prednisone. He promptly began to have more symptoms of Crohn's disease, and had to increase his prednisone again. One month later, he again reduced his prednisone, with the same result. The next month all of his Crohn's symptoms gradually disappeared. He was able to reduce his prednisone until he was off steroids. He continued on the 6-MP alone and remained well.

What Are the Side Effects?

The most worrisome side effect of all immunosuppressive

drugs is that they reduce the effectiveness of your immune system, though this is not common with the doses used for IBD. Resistance to infections decreases, which can be serious in the case of unusual infections that may be difficult to diagnose and treat. You should report any fever, chills, or persistent sore throat to your doctor promptly.

Larger doses of immunosuppressives – such as those used in transplant patients and patients being treated for certain types of cancer – increase the risk of malignancy. We still don't know whether this applies to the lower doses used in IBD. To date, no increased risk of malignancy has been shown, but we're still evaluating the data and hope to have the answer within the next few years.

The Main Immunosuppressive Drugs

Azathioprine and 6-mercaptopurine:
- used in IBD for many years;
- azathioprine is converted to 6-mercaptopurine (6-MP) in the body;
- equally effective;
- lowering of blood cell counts is reversible but occasionally life-threatening;
- pancreatitis can occur weeks after starting therapy.

Methotrexate
- available for more than 40 years, but first used in IBD in late 1980s;
- given by injection in initial studies, but well absorbed orally;
- moderately effective in Crohn's disease in 16-week study;
- long-term effectiveness unknown at present;
- benefit is expected within 2 to 12 weeks of starting therapy;

- available as tablet or injection;
- common side effects are nausea and mouth ulcers;
- no formal studies in ulcerative colitis;
- can cause cirrhosis of the liver with long-term use.

Cyclosporine

- first used in IBD in late 1980s;
- potentially severe side effects, including kidney damage, high blood pressure, liver damage;
- also causes increased facial hair and enlargement of the gums;
- risk of side effects is reduced by monitoring blood levels of drug;
- low-dose cyclosporine does not prevent flare-ups of Crohn's;
- reduces need for urgent surgery in ulcerative colitis but many patients need surgery within 6 to 12 months;
- cyclosporine enemas are not effective for ulcerative colitis;
- available as capsules, or oral or intravenous solution.

Antibiotics

Over the years, a variety of antibiotics have been used in the treatment of both ulcerative colitis and Crohn's disease. Antibiotics are not a primary therapy for ulcerative colitis, but may be given along with other forms of therapy. However, they may be used as a primary therapy in Crohn's disease, with no other medication or treatment given.

Antibiotics in Ulcerative Colitis

Antibiotics used in ulcerative colitis are generally classified as "broad spectrum." This means they are effective against a large number of different bacteria. Commonly used antibiotics in this group are ampicillin, cefazolin, gentamicin, tobramycin, ciprofloxacin, and metronidazole. Numerous other broad-spectrum antibiotics are less commonly used, mainly because they are more expensive, without added benefits.

Some gastroenterologists rarely use antibiotics in treating patients with ulcerative colitis. But doctors who do prescribe them usually use them for severe attacks. When the colon is badly inflamed, the bacteria normally present can easily penetrate the intestinal wall and move into the surrounding tissues, even the bloodstream. This can produce serious complications. Two of the most serious are septicemia (infected blood) and one or more abscesses (boils) in the liver.

Metronidazole in Crohn's Disease

The antibiotic used the most in Crohn's disease is metronidazole. It is particularly effective against a group of intestinal bacteria known as anaerobes – bacteria that do best in tissues where there is little or no oxygen.

In Crohn's disease, the full thickness of the intestinal wall is inflamed. Little breaks can develop in the inner lining of the intestine, and these breaks can lead to little openings, called sinus tracts, that penetrate through the wall of the bowel into the surrounding tissues. These sinus tracts frequently result in abscesses, and sometimes fistulas as well (see Chapter 9). Metronidazole appears to be particularly useful in the treatment of abscesses (boils) and fistulas at or near the anus. It is available as capsules or tablets, or in injectable form.

Metronidazole has been shown to benefit some patients with Crohn's colitis. Someone who has not responded to sulfasalazine may respond to metronidazole; however, someone who has not responded to metronidazole is unlikely to respond to sulfasalazine. Metronidazole is sometimes used to treat small-bowel Crohn's disease, but it has not been established to be beneficial. It may control an acute Crohn's flare-up or help suppress chronic symptoms. It does not prevent acute attacks; however, a recent study has shown that it can delay, and possibly decrease, recurrence of the disease after surgery.

There has been considerable enthusiasm for metronidazole, but no one has ever published a study comparing it with other antibiotics in the treatment of Crohn's disease. In the 1950s and 1960s tetracycline was used. The next drug to be popular was ampicillin. In the 1970s there was some enthusiasm for using erythromycin and cephalexin. Metronidazole was the drug of the 1980s. While it has continued to be popular in the 1990s, ciprofloxacin, the "new kid on the block," has also become widely used.

Side Effects of Metronidazole
By far the most common side effects of metronidazole are gastrointestinal. Nausea, decreased appetite, vomiting, constipation, diarrhea, and indigestion have all been reported, though only the first two are relatively common. Some patients complain of a constant metallic taste in the mouth. Others find that everything they eat tastes bad. The tongue may feel or even appear "furry." Continuous therapy for weeks to months can damage the nerves in the feet and legs. This shows up as persistent numbness or tingling in the feet, or difficulty with balance (clumsiness or unsteadiness), especially when walking. These effects are generally reversible, though the return to normal may take several months after the drug has been stopped.

Headaches can occur but are more likely in association with alcohol. Although most interactions with alcohol are related

---

Metronidazole and Alcohol

It was previously thought that anyone on metronidazole should avoid alcohol totally, but further experience has shown that not everyone reacts to this combination.

If you wish to drink, experiment first with very small amounts. If you want to drink beer, try just a mouthful, then two mouthfuls on another occasion, and so on. If you get to half a cup without a problem, it is very unlikely that you will experience a reaction. Try even smaller amounts of stronger drinks: a small swallow of wine or a mere sip of liquor. Many patients prefer simply to avoid alcohol rather than risk being very ill from a reaction; however, people on long-term metronidazole who hope to resume responsible drinking can minimize the risk by this gradual approach.

---

to drinking alcoholic beverages, sometimes a patient gets headaches simply by absorbing alcohol through the skin from perfumes or colognes.

Some people who drink alcohol while on metronidazole become quite ill. Symptoms include extreme flushing of the face, shortness of breath, severe headache, rapid and pounding heartbeat, nausea and vomiting, and, occasionally, collapse. Recovery is complete following a period of drowsiness or sleep.

Ciprofloxacin in Crohn's Disease

This drug is a member of a new family of antibiotics introduced within the past few years. Although no controlled studies have been done, there have been a few enthusiastic reports about this drug, alone or in combination with metronidazole, in patients with peri-anal Crohn's disease. It is also being used to treat Crohn's ileitis and/or colitis. Some centers already use it routinely despite the lack of controlled studies. One of the main drawbacks at the moment is its cost.

Side Effects of Ciprofloxacin

This drug is very well tolerated. The most common side effects are nausea and diarrhea, which occur in only about 1 in 100 patients. Ciprofloxacin slows down the inactivation of caffeine, prolonging and possibly increasing its stimulant effect. This does not mean that caffeine should be avoided, just that people who are sensitive to its stimulating effects should be aware of this possible increase. Some individuals have reported difficulty sleeping and vivid dreams. Drugs in this class can also cause inflammation of tendons (tendinitis) and there are rare reports of ruptured (torn) tendons.

Ciprofloxacin comes in tablets and there is an intravenous form, but the latter is usually unnecessary.

Other Therapies

Lidocaine Enemas

We've known for many years that chronic bowel inflammation causes enlargement of nerve cells within the bowel wall. In the past few years researchers have discovered that these nerve cells release chemicals that promote inflammation by attracting white blood cells. A few years ago, a Scandinavian doctor came up with the idea of putting local anesthetic into the rectums of people with proctitis (colitis confined to the rectum). In theory, "freezing" the nerves would prevent these chemicals from being released and would stop the inflammation. No one has had the success rates this doctor claimed, but some patients do respond to lidocaine enemas.

There is no lidocaine enema on the market, so you have to get your own enema syringe and tubes of the medication, but don't do so unless it's prescribed by your doctor. This is expensive and most drug plans don't pay for it.

When used in other ways, lidocaine can cause epileptic

seizures if absorbed into the bloodstream in large quantities. However, this side effect has not been reported with enema therapy. Other than that, there do not seem to be any side effects of using lidocaine in this way.

Topical Short-Chain Fatty Acids

Some patients with colitis limited to the left side of the colon may respond to enemas containing these naturally occurring chemicals (see Chapter 2). As with all liquid enemas, patients with colitis involving the rectum and sigmoid colon may have considerable difficulty retaining the fluid long enough to get a therapeutic effect. Other than the usual mechanical risk of having an enema, there are no side effects.

No commercial short-chain fatty-acid product exists. It is usually manufactured by hospital pharmacies at the request of a gastroenterologist, and you are charged for the cost of manufacturing as well as the ingredients. Because this is not a marketed product, drug plans do not pay for it. There is no oral form.

Cromolyn Enemas

In the mid-1970s a doctor in England reported on a group of patients with resistant ulcerative proctitis who responded to this asthma medication when it was given directly into the rectum. He noted that the rectal biopsies from these patients showed an unusually large number of eosinophils, white blood cells commonly associated with allergy. Subsequently there was some enthusiasm for using this medication in selected cases of proctitis, but it is rarely used at present.

There is no enema form. You have to purchase oral capsules, dissolve the powder in the capsules in warm water, and supply your own enema syringe.

Nicotine

Nicotine protects some people against ulcerative colitis! In the mid-1980s, the following case was reported in the medical literature.

A young woman in Boston decided to quit smoking. Shortly thereafter she developed ulcerative colitis. She was referred to a gastroenterologist but proved to have a stubborn case that did not respond well to treatment. She became frustrated and started smoking again. Her colitis got better. Once she was back to normal, she quit smoking a second time. The colitis returned and was again resistant to therapy. Once again she started smoking, and the colitis settled down. She quit smoking yet another time and the colitis returned. At this point she went to her doctor and told him that every time she stopped smoking she developed colitis, and every time she started again the colitis was controlled. Her doctor wondered if it could be the nicotine, and treated her with nicotine gum, which was the only medicinal form of nicotine available at that time. She and her doctor then determined that 12 milligrams of nicotine daily controlled her colitis, but 6 milligrams daily did not.

Statistics from the Boston university hospital system and many other centers have shown that there are three times as many nonsmokers as smokers with ulcerative colitis. Studies have also shown that it is not the act of stopping smoking that increases the risk; rather, it is simply the fact of becoming a nonsmoker. This means that a person who quits smoking has the same risk of developing colitis as a person who has never smoked.

How nicotine protects against ulcerative colitis is unknown. The therapeutic effect can be achieved by smoking but, considering the health hazards of smoking, this is obviously not a reasonable strategy. Nicotine-containing gum has been used, but is not popular because it is very sticky and hard to chew. It is better tolerated if it is sucked, but this is difficult to do for prolonged periods. The introduction of the nicotine patch has made this therapy more practical.

Nicotine patches are expensive and many drug plans will not pay for this form of treatment. People who have never smoked may be less likely to tolerate nicotine than those who have. Only brief (six-week) studies have been done. We don't know if long-term use of nicotine in this way is safe or effective. The most common side effects include nausea, light-headedness, headache, sleep disturbance or vivid dreams, dizziness, skin irritation due to the patch, sweating, and shaking of the hands.

Fish Oil
Naturally occurring chemicals known as omega-3-fatty acids have been shown to have anti-inflammatory properties. One source of these chemicals is fish oil.

A few studies have been done in ulcerative colitis and Crohn's disease, showing a modest short-term benefit. Patients who take what is considered a therapeutic amount of fish oil may end up smelling like fish! While clearly not serious, this sort of side effect is certainly undesirable. Recently, an odorless product has been produced. Further studies are needed.

Further Drugs for IBD
It is beyond the scope of this book to cover *all* the treatments for IBD described in the world literature. Some of the ones still under study are: 4-aminosalicylate (4-ASA), balsalazide, ipsalazide, prednisone metasulphabenzoate, FK-506, immuno-globulin infusions, T-lymphocyte apheresis (TLA), tumor necrosis factor (TNF), interleukins (e.g., IL-10), monoclonal antibodies, and hyperbaric oxygen.

Drugs That Reduce Symptoms without Affecting Inflammation

Certain drugs do not reduce inflammation but are used to reduce or eliminate symptoms.

Antidiarrheals

During flare-ups of IBD, most gastroenterologists prefer to avoid these drugs because complications may be more likely to occur.

But between flare-ups, many patients, especially those with Crohn's disease, are troubled by urgency, cramps, and diarrhea. The symptoms may be controlled with antidiarrheal drugs, which are generally safer than drugs that reduce symptoms by reducing inflammation.

How Do Antidiarrheal Drugs Work?

Antidiarrheal drugs work by altering the muscle activity of the small and large intestines, causing waste material to pass through more slowly.

What Are the Side Effects?

When taken between flare-ups of IBD, their main side effect is constipation, which may in turn increase abdominal pain and cause a sensation of bloating. *Do not take these drugs if you think you are having a flare-up or an obstruction, unless advised to do so by your doctor.*

The narcotic antidiarrheal medications (codeine, diphenoxylate, tincture of opium, paregoric) may also cause nausea, vomiting, drowsiness, dizziness, and itchy rashes. However, these are all very uncommon. All narcotics carry the risk of addiction, but the risk is extremely low when these drugs are used in the treatment of bowel disorders.

Loperamide is the safest of all the antidiarrheal drugs. It is chemically similar to the narcotics, but is not classified as one and is therefore available over the counter, without prescription, but it is expensive. Most drug plans will not pay for it. It is often a first choice when an antidiarrheal drug is needed. However, if cost is an issue something that is covered by drug plans may be prescribed instead.

Not only is loperamide the safest antidiarrheal drug, but it is also long-acting, so that it usually needs to be taken only once or twice a day. In comparison, diphenoxylate, codeine, and the other narcotics usually need to be taken three or four times a day. The fewer times a medication has to be taken, the more likely it is to be taken at the right times.

Loperamide is available as caplets, diphenoxylate and codeine are available as tablets, and all three are available as syrups. Tincture of opium is a liquid dosed in drops, while paregoric is a dilute solution of opium taken by the teaspoonful.

Bulk Formers

Bulk formers are drugs that bind (soak up) water in the stool, reducing looseness and sometimes frequency of stools as well. They may be thought of as commercial forms of fiber.

When are Bulk Formers Used?

Relatively mild diarrhea in both ulcerative colitis and Crohn's disease can be controlled with these products. However, bear in mind that while the stool may be more solid, it may also be more rather than less frequent.

What Are the Side Effects?

Side effects with bulk formers are very uncommon. Some individuals feel bloated and gassy. Many products give off a fine dust when they are handled; inhaling this dust repeatedly can cause you to become allergic, and serious reactions may result.

But this is extremely rare. You can avoid this by handling the products at arm's length.

Bulk formers are sold in many different flavors, as powders or granules. Most are some form of psyllium seed, a natural fiber source. Wheat bran can be equally effective.

Bile-Salt Binders

These drugs bind (form a chemical complex) with bile salts, a normal product of the liver. Bile salts flow, dissolved in the bile, from the liver via the bile duct to the intestine, where they aid in digesting fat. Normally, 90 to 99 percent of the bile salts are reabsorbed by the ileum and recycled. The 1 to 10 percent that reaches the colon is lost in the stool without causing any problems. However, if some of the ileum is diseased or has been removed, more of the bile salts reach the colon. The excess irritates the lining of the colon. This causes an outpouring of water into the colon, which is the opposite of what is supposed to happen (normally water is absorbed). The result is diarrhea. By forming a chemical complex with the bile salts, bile-salt binders can prevent this irritation.

When Are They Used?

Diarrhea in a patient with ileal disease or previous ileal resection can be treated with these drugs. However, if the diarrhea is equally well controlled by one of the other antidiarrheals, that is perfectly acceptable medically, and may well be more acceptable to the patient. These drugs are generally not used in ulcerative colitis.

What Are the Side Effects?

Patients on bile-salt binders may have difficulty digesting and absorbing fat. This occurs mainly in patients who have extensive ileal disease, or who have had a surgical resection of more than three feet (a meter) of ileum. The vitamins A, D, E, and K are all fats, and therefore may not be absorbed normally. This can generally be treated with vitamin supplements. These vitamins can be toxic; do not take them in large amounts without consulting your doctor.

Other side effects of bile-salt binders include nausea, vomiting, constipation, abdominal pain, and bloating. Occasionally folate (a B vitamin) deficiency develops due to decreased absorption. Absorption of other medications taken at the same time may be reduced or delayed.

Cholestyramine is the only antidiarrheal bile-salt binder currently available. It comes as a powder which doesn't really dissolve in anything, and it has a metallic taste. Because cholestyramine powder is inconvenient and unpalatable, many physicians (and patients) prefer to use loperamide, diphenoxylate, or codeine for diarrhea.

Drugs for Other Problems

Hemorrhoids and Anal Fissures
Hemorrhoids that are not bleeding and not causing any other problems don't require any treatment. When hemorrhoids do need to be treated, the treatment is much the same as it is for anal fissures (see Chapter 9). If bowel movements are hard, something needs to be done to make them softer. As you can imagine, the words "hard" and "soft" mean different things to different people. A misunderstanding between a doctor and a patient can lead to making the stools excessively soft. This can be a problem because excessive softening is usually associated with increased frequency, and that is often not desir-

able. As a target, you should aim for one or two large, formed, soft, easy-to-pass bowel movements every day, without forcing or straining. Many people can achieve this simply by increasing the amount of fiber in their diet.

In addition to regular bowel movements, it is useful to apply local medication to reduce inflammation in the area of the hemorrhoids and/or fissure. The things that work best are ointments and suppositories that contain a very small amount of a steroid, usually hydrocortisone. Both bowel regularity and local steroid medication shrink the tissues around hemorrhoids and reduce the overall swelling.

Reducing inflammation is a particularly important part of treating fissures. Inflammation in the region of the anus usually causes some spasm (excessive and persistent muscular activity) of the anal sphincter. This promotes constipation because passing stool is resisted. Constipation temporarily makes things better because the fissure can start to heal or hemorrhoids can start to shrink when nothing is passing through the anal canal and no attempt is being made to pass anything. However, whenever the sufferer decides to have a bowel movement the whole problem is aggravated, because forcing and straining will be necessary and the stool that comes out will be excessively hard.

Applying a steroid-containing ointment locally and regulating the stool are frequently adequate to treat hemorrhoids, but sometimes not enough to treat fissures. One of the simplest things you can do, and something that is very effective in relaxing the anal sphincter, is to use a sitz bath at least once a day. A sitz bath is a plastic bowl that looks much like a bedpan. It fits into your toilet and has a flange around it that rests on the edge of the bowl. The sitz bath has little overflow holes so that water in the pan does not spill onto the floor when you sit in it. All you need to do is fill it with plain warm water;

you don't have to add salt or baking soda. Be careful to avoid using water that is too hot, as burning the skin will simply injure and inflame it further. Five to ten minutes per sitz bath is enough. Sitz baths are best right after a bowel movement, but many people find that the most convenient time is at bedtime. If you happen to have a bidet in your bathroom, you can use it instead.

You should not use steroid-containing ointments or suppositories indefinitely, because one of the long-term side effects is a thinning of the skin, so it will actually become less resistant to irritation. Once the acute problem has subsided, continue with bowel regulation and sitz baths, as needed.

Many people are troubled by hemorrhoids or fissures as a result of chronic diarrhea rather than constipation. High-fiber diets are not usually helpful in reducing diarrhea. Your doctor is the person to consult for the best treatment of diarrhea, be it through some change in your diet or through medication.

Itching In or Around the Anus
Another complaint frequently associated with hemorrhoids is an itch in the region of the anus. This usually occurs for one or two reasons. The skin of the anal canal first becomes irritated because of frequent wiping. Once the skin is irritated, it becomes even more sensitive than usual. Stool is irritating to skin. Even when people are quite careful about wiping themselves, bits of stool are frequently left between the multiple folds of skin present in the anal canal. If you have hemorrhoids, there are even more folds where bits of stool can get trapped. The stool further inflames the already irritated skin. This results in an itch.

The treatment for an anal itch is much the same as the treatment for hemorrhoids and fissures. Controlling diarrhea is important so you won't have to wipe frequently.

What Can I Take If I Get Constipated During a Colitis Flare-up?

(For people with mild colitis involving the last two feet—about half a meter— or less of the colon)

If you have been constipated for four days or less, giving yourself a small enema of plain tapwater may be all that is necessary. An alternative is to use a suppository such as a glycerine suppository or, for something with a little more punch, a bisacodyl suppository.

If a suppository or enema does not "uncork" the system, you must generally take something by mouth to thoroughly soften and/or flush out the accumulated stool. The simplest and fastest way is to drink a bottle of a sodium-phosphate solution. Although the solution is extremely salty, the volume is so small that most people can put up with the taste for the brief time it takes to drink it. I advise my patients to mix the phosphate solution with an equal amount of sweet juice, making a total volume of about 3 ounces (100 milliliters). It is a good idea to have a glass of sweet beverage to drink right after the phosphate solution. You must drink as much clear fluid as possible – juices, broths – for the next five hours; then you can resume eating. Bowel movements will usually begin in about two hours and most people will be cleaned out within about five hours. It is not necessary to achieve the total cleanout needed before a colonoscopy or barium enema. If the attack of colitis has been con-trolled, the constipation will probably not come back. Some people cannot tolerate the extremely salty phosphate solution, while others must avoid it because it contains a lot of salt.

The second choice is to drink one or two quarts (liters) of a colonic-lavage solution. These solutions are mildly salty and contain polyethylene glycol, or PEG for short. The PEG prevents the salt and water from being absorbed into the blood and the result is that the colon is flushed out. These solutions are easier for some people to drink, though you have to take in considerably more volume than with the phosphate solution. Roughly speaking, a bottle of phosphate solution is equivalent to two liters of PEG–salt water solution.

Some patients should not or cannot drink either of these but do need something for the constipation that can occur during an attack of colitis. You should avoid harsh laxatives. This includes most over-the-counter brand-name laxatives. My suggestion (the third choice) in this situation is mineral oil. Take 2 tablespoons (30 milliliters) every two to four hours while you are awake. Eat normally. After about two days, you will usually start to pass some oil from the rectum. (You may want to put a pad or some tissue in your underwear to soak up the oil.) Continue the same dose of oil until you have had two or three large, greasy bowel movements, or ten or more smaller ones. Then reduce the oil to one tablespoon (15 milliliters) a day, in the evening, until it is clear that the attack of colitis is coming under control. At this point, you can stop the oil. The constipation should not come back.

Mineral oil is undesirable as a laxative on a regular basis. It is messy and inconvenient and it can interfere with absorption of the fat-soluble vitamins (A, D, E, and K).

It is essential that you check with your doctor before following any of these suggestions.

Cleaning the skin through the use of sitz baths is helpful because no rubbing is necessary. When you sit in the sitz bath, the anal sphincter relaxes, releasing bits of stool trapped between the folds of the anal lining. It is often helpful to apply some kind of ointment to the irritated area after the sitz bath. Initially this can be a steroid-containing ointment. Eventually what will be needed is simply something to act as a barrier to protect the skin against further irritation by stool. Zinc oxide, various baby ointments, and even petroleum jelly are all acceptable. If itching is an ongoing or frequently recurring problem, changing your toilet habits may help. After wiping off most of the residual stool following a bowel movement, fold some toilet paper, wet it, then press it onto the area around the anus. Doing this two or three times will enable you to complete cleaning the area without any rubbing. If you have diarrhea and must do this frequently, the skin will get quite dry. In this situation, apply a barrier ointment of some kind every night.

Analgesics (Painkillers)

Occasionally you may feel you need a painkiller for symptoms not controlled by your regular medications, or for some unrelated problem – a headache, for example.

ASA (aspirin in the U.S.), the most widely available non-prescription painkiller, is somewhat undesirable in IBD. Its chemical properties make ulcerative colitis patients bleed more when the colon is inflamed. Stomach and duodenal ulcers are more common in Crohn's disease patients than in the general population, and ASA increases the ulcer risk.

The preferred nonprescription analgesic is acetaminophen; it is available under many different names, but generic or "no-name" forms are just as good. Acetaminophen also has risks, but for the IBD patient it does not have as many as ASA. An overdose of acetaminophen can fatally injure the liver. Large doses taken for many years may cause kidney damage.

Nonsteroidal Anti-inflammatory Drugs (NSAIDs)

Some 10 to 20 percent of patients with IBD experience pain in one or more joints. In some cases, simple acetaminophen is enough to relieve the pain. However, many patients require drugs specifically for arthritis. Many of these fall into a family known as "nonsteroidal anti-inflammatory drugs" (NSAIDs), commonly referred to as "anti-inflammatories."

Drugs in this group include ibuprofen, naproxen, sulindac, piroxicam, ketoprofen, and diclofenac, among others.

Any of these drugs can cause inflammation of the colon (so-called NSAID colitis). This reaction is no more likely to occur in people with IBD than in those without it. It usually gets better quickly when the drug is stopped. However, there is a chance that a reaction to the drug will trigger a flare-up of the IBD. This is not an allergic reaction and it does not mean that NSAIDs must be avoided. In fact, it is not even clearly established that the same drug will cause the same reaction if it is taken again on another occasion.

Other Side Effects of NSAIDs

Up to 25 percent of patients taking NSAIDs experience burning discomfort in the upper abdomen or behind the breastbone (heartburn), or some other form of indigestion. People with a history of acid-related problems and people over 60 are much more prone to this. Other relatively common side effects are nausea and allergic reactions. The risk of ulcers in the stomach or duodenum from taking these medications can be reduced by using misoprostol at the same time, but unfortunately a common side effect of that drug is diarrhea. There is some evidence that such ulcers can be prevented by using omeprazole at the same time. The main problem with this drug is its cost.

Some NSAIDs come in slow-release forms or are long-acting and can be taken once or twice a day. Others need to be taken three or four times a day. The slow-release forms can cause ulceration and even perforation of the small intestine and colon. Because at least one of those areas is already abnormal in someone with IBD, there may be a greater risk of this happening.

Although some patients must take these drugs continuously for months or even years, using them intermittently is preferable, if possible. Most arthritis associated with IBD does not damage or destroy joints, so getting rid of the inflammation is not essential. See if you can control minor aches and pains with acetaminophen, which is considerably safer.

Antibiotics

Antibiotics are no more likely to cause adverse effects in people with IBD than in other individuals. They should be prescribed and taken when needed. But remember that antibiotics occasionally cause a form of colitis. It's usually fairly easy to distinguish between colitis due to IBD and antibiotic-associated colitis, though. If you are having an attack of colitis, always tell your gastroenterologist if you are or have been on antibiotics.

Acid-Reducing Drugs

"Heartburn," a burning sensation felt behind the breastbone or in the upper abdomen just below the breastbone, is usually due to a condition called "reflux esophagitis," in which stomach acid backs up into the esophagus. Millions of people in the world have it, including many people with IBD. The most effective therapy is to reduce the amount of acid produced by the stomach. All the drugs in this category have few side effects and can be taken with any of the standard therapies for IBD.

The best-known acid-reducing drugs are in a family known as histamine-2-receptor antagonists (also known as H-2 blockers). They include cimetidine, ranitidine, famotidine, and nizatidine.

The newest and most potent acid-suppressing medications are omeprazole and lansoprazole. However, they are also the most expensive, and are not always necessary. Stomach acid has the important protective function of killing the germs we take in with food. Therefore suppressing the production of acid just enough to relieve your symptoms is preferable.

Iron

Iron-deficiency anemia is a common problem in IBD (see Chapter 9). If it develops, most patients will require supplemental iron.

Ferrous sulfate tablets have been the standard form of iron therapy for years. However, the release of the iron from the current tablets is quite variable. Many physicians have therefore switched to ferrous gluconate as the standard iron tablet.

Common side effects of taking iron supplements are nausea and a change in bowel habit. Some people get diarrhea; others get constipated. Sometimes these side effects cause enough trouble that the dose has to be reduced or the medication even stopped. All patients on supplemental iron notice that their stools are darker, since much of the iron in each pill is not absorbed. Stools may even appear black.

If you have unacceptable side effects with even one iron tablet a day, try a combination of ferrous sulfate syrup and a high-iron diet (see below).

If you cannot get enough iron by mouth, you'll have to get it by injection, either intramuscularly (into muscle) or intravenously (into a vein). Absorption of iron from medication or food is very limited. Your doctor can monitor the need with blood tests. Do not take iron pills or high-iron foods indefinitely without your doctor's agreement.

Advantages and Disadvantages of Intramuscular Iron Injections:
- given at the doctor's office;
- should be given into large muscle mass;
- multiple injections are necessary;
- immediate side effects include pain at the injection site and allergic reactions, occasionally severe;
- risk of side effects increased if iron pills are also being taken.

Advantages and Disadvantages of Intravenous Iron Injections:
- the total dose can be given over a few hours;
- a large muscle mass is not necessary (many IBD patients are underweight);
- painless; allergy risk same as for intramuscular iron;

- possible reactions to dextran, the chemical to which iron is bound in the medication;
- must be given in hospital or clinic setting;
- unfamiliar to some doctors;
- total dose method not government-approved, but safety and efficacy are well documented.

The most important thing about receiving iron injections, either intramuscularly or intravenously, is to be sure that this form of supplementation is truly necessary.

Calcium

People on low-lactose diets may need a calcium supplement. For more information, see Chapter 5.

Other Minerals

Chronic diarrhea results in deficiencies of elements needed in trace amounts by the body. Patients who require total parenteral nutrition (see Chapter 5) are often given supplemental zinc. Occasionally, a patient will require extra chromium.

Vitamins

Many patients ask, "Do I need vitamin pills?" When the diet is restricted in some way for prolonged periods, some vitamin supplementation may be advisable. Patients on an enteral diet and those on total parenteral nutrition usually receive adequate amounts of both vitamins and minerals (see Chapter 5).

"Miracles" and Myths – The Placebo Effect

Characteristically, most chronic inflammatory diseases may get better or worse on their own. This can make any treatment look effective or ineffective. For this reason, carefully controlled studies are desirable. When patients are seriously ill,

High-Iron Foods

	Serving size	Iron (mg)
Meat and alternates		
Pork liver, cooked	3 oz (90 gm)	26.1
Beef kidney, cooked	3 oz (90 gm)	11.8
Beef, chicken liver, cooked	3 oz (90 gm)	8.0
Baked beans with pork and tomato sauce	1 cup (250 mL)	4.9
Chili with beans	1 cup (250 mL)	4.5
Corned beef	3 oz (90 gm)	3.9
Liverwurst	2 oz (60 gm)	3.2
Seeds: pumpkin, sesame	1/4 cup (50 mL)	3.2
Beef, pork, veal, ham – roasted	3 oz (90 gm)	3.0
Fruits and vegetables		
Prune juice	1/2 cup (125 mL)	5.5
Spinach (cooked)	1/2 cup (125 mL)	3.4
Cereals		
Whole-grain and dry enriched	3/4 cup (200 mL)	4.5

we cannot ethically give some of them a placebo (a substance known to have no therapeutic effect) if proven therapies are available. However, there are many situations in which temporarily withholding active treatment is acceptable, especially in the context of controlled clinical trials.

Such studies have taught us that over a four-month period 25 to 40 percent of Crohn's patients with symptoms worthy of treatment gradually get better *without* specific "active" therapy. About 20 percent of these patients remain well for one year, and 10 percent stay well for two years. In addition, many patients whose disease is brought under control *with* active therapy remain well off treatment for one or two years or more. Findings are similar for patients with ulcerative colitis.

Whenever the cause of a chronic, incurable disease is unknown, you can expect all sorts of treatments and "cures" to be promoted. Some will be touted by people who really believe in whatever they are promoting, even if they have nothing to gain. Other treatments are put forward by individuals or groups trying to "make a buck." When people are both ill and poorly informed, they may become desperate, and this makes them susceptible to being taken in.

It is important to keep the placebo effect in mind as you read the next section.

Unorthodox Therapies

Over the years, claims of dramatic success have been made for a wide variety of unorthodox therapies, sometimes on the basis of scanty reliable information.

In the 1970s, two researchers in New York maintained that a protein isolated from the pituitary gland of cows could control diarrhea in patients with Crohn's disease. In the 1980s, a company in Vermont promoted a product made from the ground-up tracheas (windpipes) of cows. In the late 1980s, two researchers in British Columbia claimed that a naturally occurring compound known as N-acetyl glucosamine was beneficial to patients with inflammatory bowel disease. Some people have asserted that patients with IBD can be greatly helped by "orthomolecular" medicine, meaning treatment with multiple vitamins and minerals.

These are just a few examples. Until the true causes of IBD are known, unorthodox treatments will continue to be promoted. We should keep an open mind about such ideas. Some may turn out to be valuable. However, because of the placebo effect, we should insist on carefully controlled, scientifically sound studies to evaluate any new proposed treatments, and view unsubstantiated claims with great suspicion. You might say, "If this has no risk, why shouldn't I try it?" Anything that has biological activity is likely also to have biological risk. The idea that avoiding standard therapies means avoiding risk is faulty. When you need treatment and you avoid it, there is a significant risk that the disease or complication will get worse, and may even endanger your life.

As I have said elsewhere in this book, by all means participate in your care. But do it in conjunction with your doctor.

SEVEN

Surgery for IBD

Many people think of surgery for inflammatory bowel disease as a last resort. Except for a few cases, it is not. Surgery is one of the important forms of treatment for IBD. Sometimes it's the best choice. Sometimes it's the only choice.

Using technical terms is unavoidable when discussing the various operations. Let's define some of the most common ones. You can also refer to the glossary at the back of the book.

In medical terminology, the suffix *-ectomy* means removal. A *colectomy* is removal of the colon. *Total colectomy* (also known as *proctocolectomy*; *procto-* from the Latin word *proctum*, which means "rectum") is removal of the colon, including the rectum. To do this, the anus must also be removed.

Another technical term for this is *abdominoperineal resection*, indicating that it is really two operations combined into one. Incisions must be made in both the abdomen and the perineum. The term *perineum* refers to the area between the anus and genitals.

Subtotal colectomy means removing all of the colon except the rectum. In the following pages, I use the term *near-total colectomy*, which means removing all of the colon and most of the rectum. It is not a standard term but is useful in explaining and understanding some of the operations.

The suffix *-ostomy* refers to a surgically created connection between a hollow organ and the skin, or between two hollow organs. *Resect* means cut out. *Anastomosis* refers to a surgically created connection. An *ileostomy* is an opening of the ileum out to the skin; a *colostomy* is the same thing using the colon. The plastic bag that fits over the opening at the skin, or *stoma* (meaning "mouth"), is called an appliance. The appliance is attached to a plastic ring that is kept in position on the abdominal wall by an adhesive paste. All ostomies, with one exception (see Kock ileostomy, below), require the wearing of an appliance.

Surgery for Ulcerative Colitis

About a third of all people with ulcerative colitis will undergo removal of the colon during their lifetime. This is for two main reasons: because medical therapy has failed to control the disease adequately; or because precancerous changes, or actual cancer, has been found in the colon.The best way to understand the various operations for ulcerative colitis is to review the history of surgery for this disease.

The 1930s and 1940s – Subtotal Colectomy, Ileostomy, and Mucous Fistula of the Rectum

In the thirties and forties, surgical techniques and peri-operative care (peri-operative refers to the time before, during, and soon after surgery) were not nearly as good as they are now. Patients undergoing a total colectomy had many complications and a significant chance of dying as a result of this surgery. The favored operation for colitis in those days was a subtotal colectomy (removal of the colon but not the rectum), with an ileostomy (artificial opening of the ileum out onto the abdomen) and a mucous fistula of the rectum (top of the rectum opening onto the abdomen). The rectum was not attached to the ileum, so the stool came out via the ileostomy.

The rectum was often severely inflamed in people having this surgery, and if the surgeon tried simply to sew up the top of the rectum, the stitches would often not hold and the contents of the rectum would leak into the abdomen – a dangerous complication. Surgeons figured out that if they brought the top of the rectum out to the skin, much like an ileostomy but smaller, such complications could be avoided. "Mucous fistula of the rectum" is the name for this procedure.

Making an Ileostomy

When ileostomies were first done, the *serosa* of the ileum was simply sewn to the skin. (The serosa is the outer lining of the intestine and is much like the tough casing around a hot dog or a sausage.) This was easy to do, but unfortunately it did not work very well. Because the body likes to close all unnatural openings, this type of ileostomy gradually became narrower and narrower in most cases. Scar tissue forms when healing takes place, and scar tissue shrinks with the passage of time. If the scar tissue is in the form of a ring – as it is in an ileostomy – when the ring shrinks, the outlet narrows. Patients would frequently develop an obstruction at the ileostomy and have to be operated on again, often more than once.

The 1950s – The Brooke Ileostomy

In 1952, a British surgeon named Bryan Brooke solved the above problem by devising what has become known as the Brooke ileostomy. Brooke figured that if the end of the ileum was folded over (much the way the end of a sleeve is folded

Brooke Ileostomy and Mucous Fistula of the Rectum

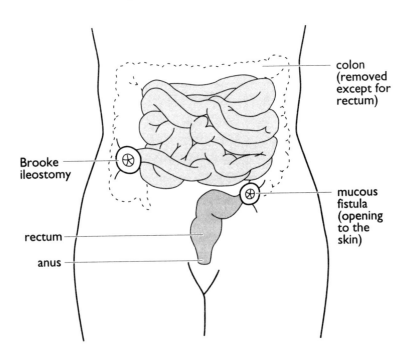

colon (removed except for rectum)

Brooke ileostomy

mucous fistula (opening to the skin)

rectum

anus

over) and *then* attached to the skin, this would usually stop the ileostomy opening from shrinking and narrowing. He was right, and the success rate for ileostomies improved dramatically. In fact, this operation has stood the test of time and is still the standard technique for creating an ileostomy.

Problems Associated with Brooke Ileostomies
Although the majority of Brooke ileostomies are trouble-free, about 25 percent of patients will have problems. Structural abnormalities can occur in and around the ileostomy, often needing surgical repair. Some people develop skin reactions to the stool, the appliance, or the adhesives. Infection with a fungus is fairly common if the skin becomes raw, but this can

be easily treated with an antifungal ointment. Leakage and odor are also possibilities that create concern. These problems can usually be treated by enterostomal therapists, nurses specializing in teaching patients about ostomies of various kinds. They are also specialists in solving various mechanical problems and skin irritation related to ostomies.

Many people with ileostomies must avoid high-roughage foods such as popcorn, nuts, sprouts, oranges, and grapefruit, or they may experience episodes of crampy abdominal pain.

As well, people with ileostomies need to pay attention to their fluid intake. Because output from the ileostomy contains more water than normal stool, not taking in enough fluids will result in less urine and an increased risk of kidney stones. You should always maintain a higher-than-normal fluid and salt intake, and be particularly careful to avoid becoming dehydrated if diarrhea occurs for any reason. A simple way to judge if you're dehydrated is to pay attention to urine output. If you have to urinate only once or twice a day and/or the volume of urine passed is small or the urine is unusually dark, you are likely dehydrated. If you urinate four or five times a day and/or urine volumes each time are large, and/or the urine is colorless or very pale yellow, dehydration is likely not a problem.

The 1950s – The Aylett Procedure

Another British surgeon, by the name of Aylett, devised a new operation in the 1950s. Aylett felt that it was unnecessary to leave people with an ileostomy. He proposed a subtotal colectomy, with anastomosis (connection) of the ileum to the rectum, so that bowel movements would occur in the normal way. He performed this operation on some 300 people and reported excellent results in about 250 of them. Unfortunately, no one else could achieve results anything like Aylett's. In the hands of most surgeons, individuals who had this type of surgery continued to have very frequent bowel movements, with great urgency and incontinence (involuntary passage of stool). As a result, the operation did not achieve widespread popularity. This operation remains a potential choice if you have ulcerative colitis with minimal rectal disease and reasonably normal rectal capacity.

The 1960s – The Kock Pouch (Kock Ileostomy, Continent Ileostomy)

In the late 1960s, a Swedish surgeon named Nils Kock came up with the idea of a continent ileostomy. "Continent" means that the patient controls the emptying of the ileostomy. (We don't refer to a Brooke ileostomy as an "incontinent ileostomy" – meaning the patient has no control over the emptying – but that's really what it is.)

Kock devised the *ileal pouch* or reservoir, which he constructed by sewing together two sections of ileum, each about 6 inches (15 centimeters) long. He determined that such a pouch would need a capacity of about 2 cups (half a liter) to act like a rectum and adequately store stool.

Kock then also devised the "nipple valve." This uses the end of the ileum to create an ileostomy that acts like a one-way valve. This valve prevents stool from coming out of the ileum on its own. When you want to empty the pouch or reservoir, you insert a tube through the nipple valve into the pouch and lean forward, and the reservoir empties through the tube into the toilet. You then pull the tube out, clean it, and put it away for next time. Individuals having this surgery have a total proctocolectomy at the same time, removing the colon and rectum.

Problems Associated with the Kock Pouch

Relatively few problems occur with this operation. The valve

A Kock Pouch and Ileostomy and Drainage of the Pouch

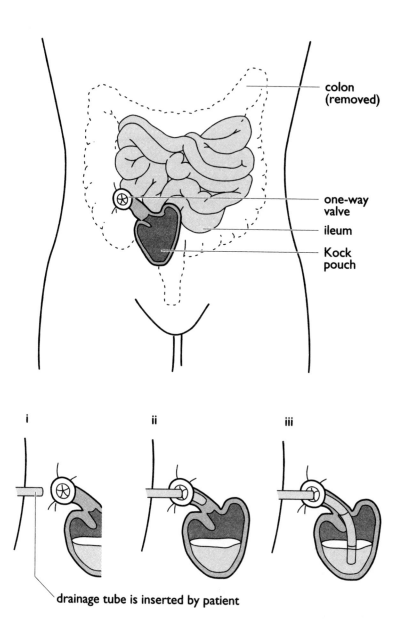

colon
(removed)

one-way
valve

ileum

Kock
pouch

i   ii   iii

drainage tube is inserted by patient

can leak enough to require wearing an appliance (ostomy bag). This can happen soon after surgery or years later. In this case, a second operation must be done to correct the valve's function. The surgical term for this is "revision" of the valve. In the early days, when many surgeons were learning the procedure, two or three revisions of the valve were often necessary, especially when the valve leaked soon after surgery. Such operations are minor, but they still require a general anesthetic.

Another common problem is inflammation of the inner lining of the pouch. Doctors seem to make up complicated-sounding names for many diseases, but this is a definite exception. The condition is simply called *pouchitis*. It is usually accompanied by loose stools, a need to empty the pouch more frequently, and, sometimes, abdominal pain. Blood may be present in the stool.

Most cases of pouchitis improve quickly with antibiotics. The most commonly used antibiotic is metronidazole (see Chapter 6).

Why Is This Operation Used for Ulcerative Colitis but Not for Crohn's Disease?

Because construction of the pouch requires about a foot (30 centimeters) of ileum, this operation is not done on people known to have Crohn's disease prior to surgery. The reason is that if Crohn's disease occurs in part of the pouch and you require surgical removal of the diseased area, then the whole pouch will have to be removed, even if the rest of it is normal. Neither doctors nor their patients like to give up any normal small bowel in Crohn's disease.

Care of the Kock Ileostomy

If you have a properly functioning Kock pouch and nipple valve, you will experience little inconvenience. Many people wear a small dressing over the ileostomy to absorb the minor amount of mucus and other intestinal fluids produced locally by the mucosa (inner lining). There are no absolute dietary restrictions, but some individuals have difficulty with indigestibles such as seeds, apple skins, and celery fibers. After you have fully recovered from surgery, there are no restrictions on activity. And there are no special problems associated with pregnancy.

If you have a Kock pouch with a continent ileostomy and are troubled by frequent pouchitis or repeated difficulties with a leaky valve, then you can have surgery and change to a Brooke ileostomy.

The Present – The Pelvic Pouch with Ileo-Anal Anastomosis
It didn't take long for surgeons to realize that Kock's idea could be combined with Aylett's, to create a pouch in the pelvis with the end of the ileum attached to the anus to allow "normal" bowel movements. This "pelvic pouch with ileoanal anastomosis" operation was introduced in the late seventies. Initially it was done by only a few specially trained surgeons. But as experience with the operation grew and statistics were collected, it gained wider acceptance and came to be the procedure of choice for most patients undergoing surgery for ulcerative colitis.

However, the operation is generally not offered to people above the age of 55 or so. The reason is that the anal sphincter muscle in older people tends to be weaker, and these individuals are much more likely to be troubled by incontinence of stool. People who have this operation at a younger age seem able to adapt better. For older patients, the best operation for ulcerative colitis is usually a total proctocolectomy and Brooke ileostomy, which requires wearing an appliance. If such a patient is ill or malnourished, or is unwell because of other

Pelvic Pouch Procedure with Ileo-Anal Anastomosis

First Stage

Brooke
ileostomy

mucous
fistula of
rectum

anus

Second Stage

loop
ileostomy

remainder
of rectum

pelvic
pouch

Third Stage

closed
ileostomy

pelvic
pouch

anus

medical conditions, the best operation is a subtotal colectomy with a Brooke ileostomy and a mucous fistula of the rectum. The rectum may be removed at a later date.

How Is the Pelvic-Pouch Operation Done?
The pelvic-pouch operation can be done as a three-stage procedure, a two-stage procedure, or a one-stage procedure. When a surgeon tells you that you are going to have a three-stage operation, you should understand that this means you are going to have three operations. It's easy to understand why surgeons prefer to say a "three-stage operation" – many people would be frightened to death if they had to think about having three operations for one problem. Nevertheless, that is actually what happens.

The Three-Stage Operation
If someone with ulcerative colitis is ill and requires surgery, it will most likely be a three-stage procedure. In the first stage you will have a subtotal colectomy, construction of a Brooke ileostomy, and a mucous fistula of the rectum. Someone in this situation will almost certainly be on steroids, and likely other medications as well. Following the operation, you will be allowed to recover and your medications will be tapered off and stopped. After an interval of three to six months, the second stage will be done. Some people are anxious to get rid of the ileostomy (and the appliance) as soon as possible. But results following the second stage are better if you have regained full health and are off most or all medications, especially steroids.

In the second stage most of the rectum will be removed, and the pelvic pouch will be constructed and connected. Strictly speaking, the ileum is not connected directly to the anus. The surgeon has to leave a very short segment of the bottom of the rectum for the end of the ileum to be attached to. Some surgeons remove the bit of mucosa (inner lining) left in this segment to totally eliminate the colitis, but most leave it in because doing so reduces the risk of incontinence.

An ileostomy will again be created. The Brooke ileostomy is also known as an "end" ileostomy, because it is made by bringing the end of the ileum out through the abdominal wall. When the pelvic pouch is created, the end of the ileum is connected to the beginning of the anus. The ileostomy created during this second operation is known as a "loop" ileostomy. With this ileostomy a hole is made in the side of the ileum and that is attached to the skin. The purpose of the loop ileostomy, which is temporary, is to divert stool before it gets down to the pouch and ileo-anal anastomosis. The reason is to create the best possible conditions for this complex surgery to heal. This process of healing generally takes two to three months.

You will then return for the third stage of the procedure. This is a minor operation, but it still requires a general anesthetic. Here the loop ileostomy is closed so that you can begin having bowel movements "the normal way."

If you are not particularly ill, this three-stage operation can be combined into two stages. In the first stage, you will have a near-total colectomy and the pelvic pouch, the ileo-anal anastomosis, and the loop ileostomy will be created. About three months later, the loop ileostomy will be closed.

At the beginning of the 1990s, IBD surgeons began experimenting with doing the entire operation in one stage. While this is appealing, the results to this point have not been as good. More patients have postsurgical complications than those with the temporary loop ileostomy. With further experience and further improvements in technique perhaps the one-stage operation will become commonplace, but at this point it is not recommended for most patients.

Side Effects and Complications of Pelvic-Pouch Surgery
This surgery involves the risk of several side effects and complications.

Frequent and/or urgent bowel movements: Pelvic-pouch surgery allows you a return to health, but most people still have an average of 3 to 5 semiformed bowel movements a day. This varies considerably – some people have 10 to 12 a day. Many are much better off taking regular doses of either loperamide or diphenoxylate (see Chapter 6), with supplemental doses as necessary. Even without antidiarrheal drugs, urgency is not a problem for most patients.

Incontinence: If someone with a pelvic pouch has frequent, unpredictable bowel movements, with episodes of incontinence, little has been achieved, even though the colitis is cured. Initially many people have quite frequent stools and some degree of urgency. A small number of patients are troubled by incontinence during the day. A somewhat larger number are troubled by incontinence that occurs only at night. The reason for this difference is that all people pass gas from the rectum while asleep. If there is less-than-normal sensitivity in the anal canal, and particularly if loose stool is present, the gas may be accompanied by a small amount of fluid without you being aware of it. Many patients wear a pad at night; only a few need to wear one during the day. Some patients have more than a little incontinence of stool, and this is a major problem.

Fortunately, a significant degree of adaptation occurs during the first three to six months following the operation. The pouch gets larger and "learns" to store stool, acting like a rectum. As this happens, the daily number of trips to the bathroom decreases, and incontinence also decreases. Still, many patients continue to wear a pad at night for psychological comfort, even after the incontinence is gone.

If incontinence remains a major problem, there is usually

little choice but to give up the pelvic pouch and have another operation. You can then have a Kock ileostomy; or, to have the best chance of not needing any further surgery, you can simply have a Brooke ileostomy.

Pouchitis: Whether you have a Kock pouch higher up in the abdomen in combination with a continent ileostomy or a pelvic pouch with an ileo-anal anastomosis, pouchitis (inflammation of the pouch) is the second most common problem. Most cases respond well to antibiotics. Persistent pouchitis raises the possibility of Crohn's disease.

Sexual dysfunction: Most people report that sexual function is unchanged or improved following surgery. Improvement usually reflects better general health. However, of men having this surgery, 1 to 2 percent become impotent or are unable to reach orgasm after surgery; about 4 percent experience retrograde ejaculation, which means that the semen goes into the bladder instead of coming out of the penis. In women, frequency of intercourse and ability to reach orgasm tend to increase after surgery, and painful intercourse decreases. No sex-specific problems have been reported in women after surgery.

Narrowing of the anastomosis: Any time tissue is cut and then sewn or stapled together, a certain amount of scar tissue forms. Some people make more scar tissue than others. Scar tissue tends to shrink with the passage of time. If the scar tissue encircles a tube, then shrinkage of the scar tissue may produce narrowing.

In about 5 percent of patients undergoing ileo-anal anastomosis, a stricture (narrowing) develops at the site of the anastomosis. This can usually be treated by dilatation (stretching), which is a simple procedure done with a local anesthetic and/or sedative, but usually not requiring a general anesthetic.

Postoperative leak: Postoperative leak happens occasionally

Who Can Have a Kock Pouch and Ileostomy?

The Kock (continent) ileostomy is an alternative to the Brooke ileostomy for certain ulcerative colitis patients in the following groups:

- those with a Brooke ileostomy who have had a total proctocolectomy and who wish to avoid wearing an appliance;
- those who need a colectomy but are not candidates for a pelvic pouch, usually because of poor anal-sphincter function;
- those who prefer a continent ileostomy to a pelvic pouch with ileo-anal anastomosis – usually patients who cannot make frequent trips to the bathroom because of their jobs;
- those who have had a failed ileo-anal anastomosis but still prefer continence to wearing an external appliance.

with any type of bowel surgery, and does not reflect badly on the surgeon. If a leak occurs, an abscess (boil) is likely to form next to the anastomosis. This will result in pain in the pelvis or around the anus, and fever. The abscess will generally require drainage, either by inserting a very fine needle into it to extract the pus, or by making a small cut into the abscess with a scalpel so the pus can drain on its own. Sometimes infection due to a leak will clear up simply with antibiotic therapy.

Inflammation at the anastomosis: Because many people are left with a tiny piece of rectal lining, it is possible to have persistent or recurrent colitis in this area. Thus far it has not been a problem in most patients. When it occurs, it is usually treated with 5-ASA or hydrocortisone suppositories.

Cancer: Cancer of the colon occurs more commonly in people with ulcerative colitis than it does in the general population. When the whole colon is removed (total proctocolectomy), the risk is removed. When a person undergoes a pouch procedure with an ileo-anal anastomosis, a tiny amount of colon (the last bit of the rectum) is left in. Even if the surgeon peels off whatever can be seen of the inner lining of the colon during surgery, it is always possible that a few microscopic glands will be left behind. These glands could at some point give rise to a cancer. With the shift to leaving the mucosa (inner lining) intact, the risk is slightly greater, but overall it is still extremely low.

Indeterminate Colitis

We are unable to distinguish ulcerative colitis from Crohn's disease in about 10 percent of patients. In most centers, if surgery is needed, such patients are given the benefit of the doubt and are offered a pelvic-pouch procedure with ileo-anal anastomosis. However, patients should understand that the chances that this operation will fail are higher than they are for patients with "clearcut" ulcerative colitis. Still, the chances of success are reasonably good. If the problem is in fact ulcerative colitis, the failure rate will be no more than usual. If it is Crohn's disease, there is still a better than 50 percent chance the procedure will be successful.

Surgery for Crohn's Disease

Surgery for ulcerative colitis involves removing most or all of the colon. Surgery for Crohn's disease depends on where in the GI tract the disease occurs.

People with Crohn's disease require surgery for three main reasons: the failure of medical therapy to control the disease adequately; chronic or frequently recurring obstructions; and abscesses with or without fistulas (abnormal channels).

The decision that medical therapy has failed to control the disease adequately, and that surgery is needed, should be made jointly by the gastroenterologist, the surgeon, and the patient (or patient's parents). The criteria may be different for different people.

Thickening of Intestinal Wall

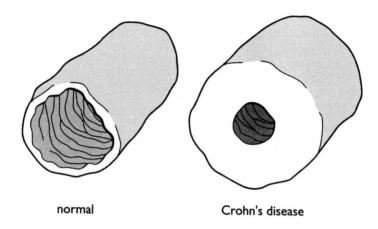

normal   Crohn's disease

Obstructions

You can think of the intestine as an elastic band. It has a thin wall; the opening is large in relation to the thickness of the wall, and it is able to stretch easily. When Crohn's disease occurs in the intestine, the wall becomes swollen. It swells outward, but it also swells inward. Now the intestine is more like a tire. It is still somewhat stretchy, but the wall is thicker and stiffer and the channel is much narrower.

During an acute episode, the swelling increases even more. The wall swells outward more (which is not a problem) but it also swells inward more. The intestinal channel does not have to be completely blocked to act blocked. If a patient with acute small-bowel obstruction goes on a clear-fluid diet or takes prednisone, the swelling will almost always decrease and the obstruction will get better, usually within 48 hours.

If a patient begins to have frequently recurring obstructions or has some symptoms of obstruction all the time (nausea, bloating, and crampy abdominal pain soon after every meal), the narrowing of the intestine is likely due not only to swelling, but also to scarring. Steroids or an enteral (sterilized liquid) diet should reduce the swelling. But when the narrowing is due mainly to scarring, no drug or diet treatment will relieve the problem for long.

An area of scarring may be dilated (stretched) with an inflatable balloon passed through an endoscope, if the area can be reached with a scope. But most doctors agree that only about 20 percent of patients, at most, experience relief for a substantial period of time (more than a year). Eventually surgery is necessary.

There are two types of surgery: strictureplasty and resection. *Strictureplasty* comes from *stricture*, meaning narrowing, and *-plasty*, meaning shaping something through the use of surgery. You can think of the procedure as plastic surgery on the intestine. *Resection* means removing something by cutting it out.

The idea in strictureplasty is to take a narrowed area of intestine and make it wider. Patients with Crohn's disease of the small bowel who should be considered for this type of surgery fall into two groups: those who have had a previous resection and need another operation, and those who need surgery and have never had it before, but have very extensive disease. Some people undergoing strictureplasty also require resection (removal) of additional segments of diseased tissue that are not suitable for strictureplasty.

Most people who undergo strictureplasty are later able to stop taking most or all medications, eat normally, and gain weight. In long-term follow-up, the majority of strictures that are opened in this way remain open. When people who have had strictureplasty require surgery for obstruction again, it is usually due to the formation of new strictures.

What is interesting about this surgery is that the Crohn's

Strictureplasty

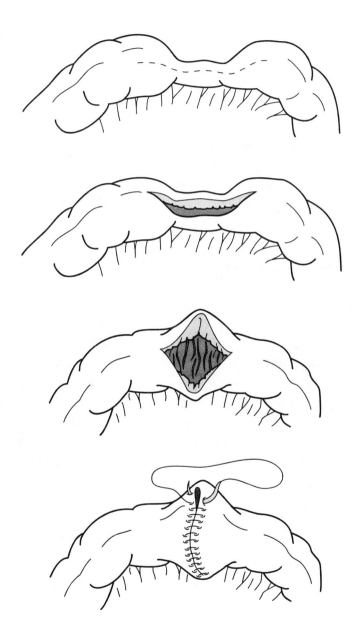

disease in the area of the operated-on stricture seems to improve considerably after the operation. When strictureplasty patients are operated upon for some other reason, the areas of strictureplasty usually appear much less inflamed than before the strictureplasty. We can conclude that, while the disease itself causes the narrowing, the narrowing somehow makes the disease worse.

Surgery for Crohn's of the Ileum
Although Crohn's disease is often referred to as a segmental or patchy disease, in most people the disease occurs at the end of the ileum, with or without involving the beginning of the colon. When such people require surgery for the first time, they have a resection of the area of the disease with anastomosis (connection) of the new end of the ileum to the ascending colon in one of two ways. This is generally a simple, straight-forward operation. It's just like cutting out the middle of a shirtsleeve and sewing the lower end to the upper end.

Some people having a resection have one or more fistulas from the area of disease to another part of the bowel which is not affected by Crohn's disease. The surgeon may have to remove a little piece of bowel where the fistula runs in. If you have such a fistula and it leads to the rectum, you may need a temporary colostomy to divert the stool away from site of the repaired fistula, allowing the rectum to rest and heal properly. In a minor operation, the colostomy will be closed two to three months later.

Common Side Effects of Resection of the End of the Ileum
Removing the end of the ileum is not without consequences. These include:

- *Diarrhea due to loss of the ileocecal valve:* The ileocecal

Surgery for the Most Common Form of Crohn's Disease

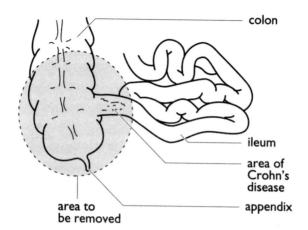

colon

ileum

area of Crohn's disease

appendix

area to be removed

end-to-side

side-to-side

valve allows liquid intestinal contents to be discharged into the colon in a controlled, intermittent fashion. Surgical removal can lead to diarrhea. This effect is almost always temporary.

- *Bile-salt diarrhea*: Normally, 90 to 99 percent of bile salts reaching the ileum are recycled back to the liver and reused. The remaining 1 to 10 percent are lost into the colon. When even a bit of ileum is removed, the amount lost each day into the colon is increased.

  Certain bile salts have a laxativelike effect on the colon, and the colon loses salt and water instead of absorbing them as it is supposed to. The result is diarrhea. Fortunately, bile-salt diarrhea is usually easy to control with drugs (see Chapter 6).

- *Decreased fat digestion and absorption*: When you undergo resection (removal) of more than about a yard (a meter) of the end of the ileum, two things happen. First, the liver is unable to maintain a normal level of bile salts in the intestine to digest fat. Second, large resections such as this interfere with absorption of the fat that is digested, because fat requires the greatest length of intestine for its absorption.

  If cholestyramine is being used to treat bile-salt diarrhea, that drug will further reduce the quantity of available bile salts and this will further interfere with fat digestion and, indirectly, with fat absorption. Unabsorbed fat is broken down by bacteria in the colon, producing chemicals that have a laxative effect and possibly aggravating the diarrhea. Fortunately, a relatively small number of patients end up having more than a yard of ileum removed, even when they require a second or third resection.

- *Decreased vitamin B$_{12}$ absorption:* Another function of the ileum is to absorb vitamin B$_{12}$. If more than about 18 inches (45 centimeters) of ileum is removed, you will likely have subnormal vitamin B$_{12}$ absorption. If this is the case, no amount of swallowed B$_{12}$ will fix the problem, since there is simply not enough ileum available for absorption. The intestine may adapt somewhat in the first six months after resection. About six months after the resection, it is generally a good idea to have a Schilling test, to determine whether B$_{12}$ absorption is normal or not. It has no risks and is very accurate.

  For the Schilling test, you are given an injection of B$_{12}$ and then asked to drink a radioactive B$_{12}$ fluid (don't worry; there's no danger!) Then you collect your urine for two days – in a separate container for each day – and the radioactivity is measured to indicate the amount of B$_{12}$ that your body absorbed.

  Some doctors simply put their patients on B12 shots after resection of a piece of ileum. However, these injections go on once a month – forever. It is well worth going through a Schilling test to determine if this is really necessary before you make a pincushion out of yourself. If you do not go on regular injections, your blood level of B12 should be measured intermittently. For some patients it is easier and simpler to take the injections, without having the Schilling test.

Surgery for Jejunal Crohn's Disease

Most jejunal disease is treated by resection, but some patients undergo strictureplasty. The ileum is able to compensate completely for the loss of the jejunum, even with extensive resections.

Surgery for Crohn's Colitis

Location of disease	Possible operations	Advantages	Disadvantages
Most or all of colon (including rectum)	• Total proctocolectomy & Brooke ileostomy	• Lowest chance of recurrence	• Perineal incision, which may not heal completely
	• Subtotal colectomy, Brooke ileostomy, oversewn rectum	• No perineal incision	• Risk of persistent or recurrent disease in rectum • Access to rectum for cancer checkup may be difficult
Most or all of colon but normal rectum	• Total proctocolectomy & Brooke ileostomy	• Lowest chance of recurrence	• Perineal incision • Need for appliance
	• Subtotal colectomy, Brooke ileostomy, oversewn rectum	• No perineal incision	• Risk of persistent or recurrent disease in rectum • Need for appliance • Access to rectum for cancer checkup may be difficult
	• Subtotal colectomy & ileorectal anastomosis	• No perineal incision • No need for appliance	• Highest chance of recurrent disease in ileum or rectum • Need for cancer surveillance of rectum • Frequent bowel movements

Location of disease	Possible operations	Advantages	Disadvantages
Short segment (excluding rectum)	• Segmental resection	• Low chance of diarrhea • Simple operation	• High chance of recurrent disease
Rectum only	• Colostomy only	• Simple operation	• Need for appliance • Possible persistent or recurrent rectal or peri-anal disease
	• Colostomy and proctectomy	• Better chance of prolonged relief of symptoms	• Perineal incision • Need for appliance
Ileum and colon	• Selective, if symptoms are distinctively ileum *or* colon	• Conserves bowel (fewer side effects)	• Higher recurrence rate

Surgery for Duodenal Crohn's Disease

A few people develop narrowing of the lumen (channel) in the duodenum, so that food cannot pass. Resection or stricture-plasty surgery is technically difficult because of the duodenum's anatomic location. The simplest and safest approach is a bypass operation called a "gastrojejunostomy." In this operation, a loop of upper jejunum is surgically attached (anastomosed) to the stomach. Several side effects may occur, but they are beyond the scope of this book.

Surgery for Crohn's Disease of the Stomach

People with Crohn's of the stomach rarely require surgery. If they do, it is mainly because of narrowing and obstruction of the lower third of the stomach. The usual operation is a gastrojejunostomy, as described above.

Surgery for Crohn's Disease of the Esophagus

Esophageal Crohn's disease is extremely rare. Part or all of the esophagus (swallowing tube) can be removed, if necessary. Some surgeons simply pull the stomach up into the chest and connect it to the remaining esophagus. Others use a section of the patient's jejunum or colon to bridge the gap.

Surgery for Crohn's Disease of the Colon (Crohn's Colitis)

Surgery for Crohn's disease of the colon varies according to how much of the colon is involved, how severe the disease is, what the surgeon and gastroenterologist advise, and what the patient or the patient's family wants. The common reasons for surgery for Crohn's colitis are the same as for Crohn's disease in general: failure of medical therapy to control the disease adequately, abscesses with or without fistulas, and obstructions.

Side Effects of Surgery for Crohn's Colitis

After small segments of the colon are surgically removed, bowel habits should generally be normal. But since the function of colon is to remove water from the stool, the more colon is lost, the more likely it is you will have diarrhea. This can often be controlled with antidiarrheal drugs.

Side Effects of Ostomies with the Rectum Left in Place

Some of the stool consists of mucus, living and dead bacteria, and dead lining cells of the bowel. Even if the rectum is disconnected, it continues to produce mucus, provide a home for bacteria, and shed its lining regularly. In other words, it continues to make stool!

Although there is no food residue, the stool that is made accumulates and must be emptied every so often. Some patients make more; others make less. But everyone who has a disconnected rectum will continue to have the urge to have a bowel movement in the normal way every so often. Some patients, particularly those who have not been warned, are confused when they get the urge to go to the toilet. "I must be going crazy. My rectum is disconnected from my intestines but I still feel I have to have a bowel movement!" Of course they're not crazy. They are getting the urge to pass the nonfood portion of the stool.

You shouldn't resist the urge. If you do, the stool will accumulate. Just like normal stool that is held in, the stool will get drier and drier and harder and harder. It will accumulate until the rectum fills up. When that happens, you will generally start to get increasing pressure and discomfort in the pelvic region. Sooner or later you'll see a doctor, who will examine you and find that the rectum is full. Some patients find it necessary to give themselves a small enema every so often.

Recurring Crohn's Disease After Surgery

The chance of Crohn's disease coming back after surgery is highest if you have combined small-bowel and colon disease, slightly lower if you have pure small-bowel disease, and lowest if you have pure colon disease, provided you have had all of the colon removed or all of the colon except for the rectum. Just to make things more confusing, there are three different kinds of recurrence referred to in the medical literature. One kind is *endoscopic* recurrence – that is, recurrent disease that is found by examining your bowel with a scope. European researchers have demonstrated that many people undergoing small-bowel resection have evidence of new disease in the ileum visible with the colonoscope within 12 weeks of surgery; however, the vast majority of these patients will not have symptoms at that time. Another kind of recurrence is what is of concern to most patients – a return of symptoms and signs of the disease. The third type of recurrence is the need for further surgery. Despite numerous studies, we have little knowledge about the factors that influence recurrent Crohn's disease. Recent evidence has suggested that smoking increases the risk.

For individuals with pure small-bowel disease or those with combined small-bowel and large-bowel disease, most recurrences will be in the ileum, starting from the anastomosis (connection) and extending upward. Why it is much less common for the disease to recur downstream from the anastomosis is just one more mystery of Crohn's disease. The symptoms, signs, and extent of disease prior to surgery cannot be used to predict the symptoms, signs, and extent when the disease comes back.

Current figures suggest that about 15 to 25 percent of patients with small-bowel disease (with or without colonic disease) will have symptoms of the disease within two years of surgery, 30 to 50 percent within about five years, and about 70 percent within ten years. It is believed that, if patients lived long enough, the recurrence rate of small-bowel Crohn's would be 100 percent.

For disease of the colon the situation is not so clear. If a patient has a short segment of diseased colon removed, there is probably a 75 percent chance of developing further disease. But if the entire colon plus rectum is removed, some centers suggest that the recurrence rate in the ileum will be as low as 10 percent, while other equally authoritative centers suggest that the risk is as high as 40 percent. There is also a higher risk of recurrent Crohn's disease in the ileum in patients who undergo subtotal colectomy and ileorectal anastomosis than in those with subtotal colectomy and ileostomy.

One of the reasons the statistics on surgery for Crohn's

colitis are so confusing is that far fewer patients require surgery, compared with people who just have Crohn's disease of the ileum, or ileum and colon. So in any given center for IBD there may not be enough patients to provide statistically meaningful numbers about the outcome of a particular operation.

Looking at Crohn's disease overall, without regard to where the disease occurs, various studies have suggested that the chance of you needing any surgery for Crohn's disease is about 80 percent. The chance of you needing a second operation after a first resection is 25 to 40 percent at 5 years, 30 to 60 percent at 10 years, and 40 to 70 percent at 20 years.

Surgical Treatment for Abscesses and Fistulas

About 25 percent of patients with Crohn's disease are troubled by what is referred to as "peri-anal disease," which literally means disease around the anus. The problems that usually require surgery include abscesses (boils) and fistulas (see Chapter 9).

How Does an Abscess Form?

Abscesses and fistulas in Crohn's disease arise because of little breaks in the inner lining of the small or large intestine. These breaks in the lining allow germs (such as bacteria) that are normally present in the rectum to get into the tissues (such as the mesentery or the tissues around the rectum), where they shouldn't be. This is referred to as a "confined perforation." The presence of the germs triggers a response by the body that is just like a country responding to an invading force. The body sends in white blood cells (the army) to attack the bacteria. The white cells kill some bacteria and the bacteria kill some white cells. Initially, the white cells win. However, once the break in the lining lets germs exit from the small bowel or colon, it almost always stays open. The result is that bacteria continue to enter the tissues, and this leads to a continuing infection, a continuing response by the body, and a continuing presence of white blood cells. The result is the gradual accumulation of pus, which is a mixture of living and dead white cells and living and dead germs. Common examples of pus in everyday life are the yellow or green stuff that comes out of your nose when you have a bad cold or the greenish yellow substance that appears on the surface of your skin a few days after you suffer a bad scrape.

When you initially have an abscess, you don't feel anything. But gradually the accumulating pus puts pressure on the adjacent tissues. Sooner or later, the infection results in swelling and pain, and possibly a fever as well.

How Is an Abscess Treated?

The treatment for a collection of pus is to drain it. Sometimes the body will cause the drainage to occur without a doctor having to do anything. Think of having an acne pimple on your forehead. As the pimple grows, it becomes more and more uncomfortable because the skin around the pimple is being stretched due to the pressure of the pus within it. Many people with a painful acne pimple will squeeze it because they know that this will pop a little hole in the surface of the skin, most of the pus will drain out, and the pain will go away. A somewhat more pleasant way of accomplishing the same thing is to apply warm wet compresses to the area. This will soften the skin and make it easier for the pimple to spring a leak and drain itself.

An abdominal or peri-anal abscess is really just like a giant pimple. If the abscess bulges toward the surface of the abdomen or buttock, it may drain spontaneously. If you soak the area (by taking sitz baths, if it is a peri-anal abscess) this will encourage drainage. The skin in the area of the abscess softens and the pressure inside the abscess may cause it to break open and drain.

How an Abscess Forms in Crohn's Disease

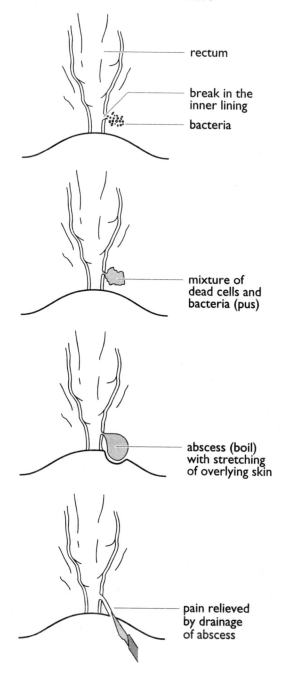

rectum

break in the inner lining

bacteria

mixture of dead cells and bacteria (pus)

abscess (boil) with stretching of overlying skin

pain relieved by drainage of abscess

Unfortunately, an abscess must often become quite large before it bulges the surface of the skin, and this means that it can become quite painful. Many patients cannot tolerate the pain while waiting for an abscess to drain spontaneously. Indeed, they should not wait – occasionally people become quite ill. At a hospital or doctor's office the abscess can be drained by freezing the area and making a small hole with a scalpel or a needle through the skin directly into the abscess. If a peri-anal abscess is large, you may have to be taken to the operating room and given a general anesthetic so a surgeon can adequately drain it. Large abdominal abscesses are almost always easily drained with the aid of ultrasound or CAT scan guidance.

Draining the abscess does not always end the problem in patients with Crohn's disease. In most patients, the little opening in the inner lining of the intestine that led to the abscess remains, as we've said. After drainage of the abscess, the result is a connection between the inside of the intestine and the outside world via the skin. This is one example of a fistula.

If a peri-anal abscess does not point toward the skin but points and presses instead on the patient's bladder, it may drain spontaneously into the bladder. This will solve the immediate problem of the abscess, but the person will be left with a fistula to the bladder that will require treatment. The same situation can occur if the abscess points toward and pushes on the vagina. If a fistula to the bladder, vagina, or skin surface in a location other than the perineum is treated surgically, removal of the piece of intestine that is the source of the fistula is usually necessary. Some fistulas simply connect two segments of intestine; often nothing needs to be done about these.

Sometimes multiple breaks in the lining occur close together. This may result in a large mass of inflamed tissue containing many little abscesses, called a "phlegmon." Treatment for this

Fistulous Tract with Chronic Abscess

i

rectal wall

chronic abscess

surgical incision

ii

gauze packing

iii

fistulous tract
(often remains open)

scar tissue lining tract

condition is almost always surgical resection of the segment of intestine that is the source of infection.

Treatment of a Chronic Abscess

Many patients with peri-anal abscesses can be treated with sitz baths and antibiotics, but some need surgery. In some cases the surgeon must create a wedge-shaped opening into the abscess to clean it out thoroughly. Afterward, the wound cavity may be packed with gauze, which is usually changed daily. If this is not done, the wound usually closes over at the surface faster than it does deeper down, so that the abscess cavity remains and becomes filled with pus again. The packing keeps the skin wound open so that the wound heals from the bottom up (or, to put it another way, from the inside out).

If the procedure is totally successful, the area heals completely, leaving a scar. However, in most cases the patient is left with a fistulous tract, which is a narrow, straight, tubelike path from the inside of the bowel out to the skin, without an abscess cavity. Drainage is usually a relatively minor problem and most people can put up with it.

Unfortunately, those people who develop peri-anal fistulas often get other abscesses and fistulas and need surgery again.

Adhesions

Any time a patient has surgery on the GI tract, bands of scar tissue are going to develop afterward. These bands, known as adhesions, will run from the point of surgery to other segments of intestine, to other organs, or to the peritoneum (lining of the abdominal cavity), particularly at the site of the previous incision. In most people they do not cause any problems. Adhesions don't hurt. What they can do is fix the intestine at a certain point so that, if it becomes twisted, an obstruction will occur. Most such obstructions get better without surgical

What Is a Fistula?

A fistula is an abnormal connection between a hollow structure (such as the rectum) and the skin surface or between two hollow structures such as two loops of bowel, or bowel and bladder, or bowel and vagina. The path that the fistula follows is referred to as a "fistulous tract," and may be short or quite long.

Peri-anal Fistula

Recto-vaginal Fistula

Ileo-vesical (Ileum-to-bladder) Fistula

treatment. However, some people need surgery to untwist the bowel and cut the adhesions. Of course, new adhesions will form, but usually they will not cause trouble.

EIGHT

Children with IBD

Both ulcerative colitis and Crohn's disease can begin at any age. However, ulcerative colitis is rare in infancy, while Crohn's disease is not unusual. Fifteen percent of patients with ulcerative colitis develop it before the age of 20, whereas in Crohn's disease the figure is 25 to 30 percent.

Recent research has suggested that second-hand smoke increases the risk of inflammatory bowel disease, particularly Crohn's disease, in children. One study showed a possible increased risk of ulcerative colitis as well, even though smoking seems to protect against ulcerative colitis in adults (see Chapter 2).

Diagnosing IBD in Children

Many aspects of ulcerative colitis and Crohn's disease in children are identical to those in adults, but there are some important differences. The symptoms of both diseases seem to be more pronounced in children than in adults. There is also some evidence that children have more intestinal complications (see Chapter 9). However, they have fewer nonintestinal problems than adults.

Most children with ulcerative colitis are diagnosed fairly promptly, because blood is found in the stool. The diagnosis of Crohn's disease, however, is often delayed. Previously, the time between the onset of symptoms and a diagnosis of Crohn's disease averaged 3 years. This has decreased in the past 20 years because of greater awareness of the disease.

Many children with Crohn's develop the typical crampy abdominal pain, diarrhea, and weight loss, but some have only a low-grade fever with few other symptoms. Sometimes it's hard to tell what's going on. Many otherwise normal young children suffer from abdominal pain related to lactose intolerance or constipation, and some children complain about abdominal pain that is a result of emotional stress. Poor appetite and weight loss can lead to an erroneous diagnosis of anorexia nervosa. In some children, the only sign of Crohn's initially is a failure to grow; parents and doctors are alerted by the child's small size or delayed puberty.

The Issue of Growth

Even after an accurate diagnosis is made, growth failure in children with IBD is a concern. However, we've learned a lot in the past 20 years. We used to think that using glucocorticoids to treat the disease was a major factor in delayed growth. The bulk of the evidence now suggests that the major factor is how active the disease is. The more severe the disease, and the longer the time it is active, the more growth will be delayed, even prevented. Glucocorticoids may play some role in delayed growth, but growth is likely to improve if the drugs suppress the disease so the child will eat better.

Drug Therapy for Children with IBD

Generally children receive the same drugs as adults, but the doses of some need to be adjusted to body weight, and a few drugs are avoided because they can interfere with the development of certain tissues. Because IBD is more aggressive in children, steroids are given more frequently to them than to adults.

Extra Nutrition for Children with Crohn's

Researchers in Montreal have been leaders in demonstrating that some children with Crohn's disease will grow more if their normal diet is supplemented with nightly feeds of a liquid diet (see Chapter 5). In fact, many children learn to slip small feeding tubes through their noses down into their stomachs each night at bedtime. A bag of enteral (sterilized liquid) diet is hung on a pole and dripped into the tube while the child is asleep. In the morning, the child pulls out the tube and has a normal day. A thousand or more extra kilocalories (4,184 kilojoules) can be taken in this way.

Surgery for Children with IBD

Obviously, the most effective way to reduce inflammation is to remove it surgically. Indeed, doctors tend to be somewhat more aggressive about treating children surgically, because of the concern about growth, and also because the IBD tends to be more aggressive. Nevertheless, unless puberty has already begun, there is a span of several years in which to suppress the disease and allow growth. No one should jump to the conclusion that children should immediately undergo surgery because their growth is delayed. Not all children with IBD will grow simply because they have surgery; they may just be naturally short.

Psychological Effects of IBD on Children

Children – particularly teenagers – are very anxious not to be seen as different from their peers; their self-consciousness, and the intolerance of other children, often leads to a degree of isolation.

Most children, like most adults, become tough as a result of having a chronic disease. But this takes time. Parents must try to treat these children the same way they treat their other children. Whenever possible, children with IBD should be allowed to participate in normal activities. Unnecessary dietary restrictions should be avoided. For example, there is no evidence that people with IBD need to avoid "junk foods."

It is natural to feel depressed when IBD is diagnosed or when it flares up. Many kids think, "Why me?" However, once treatment begins and the symptoms subside, most will perk up. During a flare-up, extra rest *may* be necessary. When improvement comes, regular activities *may* have to be resumed gradually.

It is desirable for the child to establish a comfortable relationship with the doctor. Family, close friends, and, at times, other patients can be a big help, but the doctor-patient relationship remains extremely important.

NINE

Complications of IBD

Complications are unforeseen conditions that occur during the course of a disease. Sometimes they arise before the disease is diagnosed, and serve as symptoms or signs that lead a physician to the disease.

The complications of IBD can be divided into two types: those related to the intestine itself, and those outside the intestine. Here are some of the more common ones.

Complications in the Intestine

Toxic Megacolon

From a medical viewpoint the most severe complication of any type of colitis is toxic megacolon. The word "toxic" means that the patient is acutely ill with fever, abdominal pain, loss of appetite, diarrhea, nausea, and possibly vomiting. "Megacolon" refers to the fact that part or all of the colon is abnormally wide in diameter.

In this condition, the muscular wall of the colon becomes more or less paralyzed. As a result, the gas normally produced by the bacteria in the colon accumulates instead of passing out the rectum. Toxic megacolon is the most feared complication of colitis mainly because it is sometimes associated with perforations (holes) in the wall of the colon. The contents of the bowel (including bacteria) can leak into the abdominal cavity, resulting in *peritonitis*, a condition in which the lining of the abdominal wall is inflamed. This is a very serious, sometimes fatal illness. The perforations require emergency surgery. The usual operation is subtotal colectomy, Brooke ileostomy, and mucous fistula of the rectum (see Chapter 7).

If there is no evidence of perforation, standard treatment is steroids, but surgery is often necessary.

Toxic megacolon can occur with both ulcerative colitis and Crohn's disease. It is less common in Crohn's colitis because, as the disease progresses, the colon wall becomes thick, scarred, and less likely to stretch. Toxic megacolon is more common in people who have extensive colitis than it is with colitis limited to a relatively small segment of the colon.

Strictures

Both ulcerative colitis and Crohn's disease can be complicated by strictures, or localized areas of narrowing. Strictures are much more common in Crohn's disease than in ulcerative colitis, because Crohn's causes inflammation of the full thickness of the wall of the bowel. Ulcerative colitis generally involves only the inner lining.

Strictures may lead to bowel obstruction, which may be temporary (acute) or permanent (chronic). Bowel obstruction is the most common complication of small-bowel Crohn's disease. It can occur suddenly or gradually. Sudden or acute obstruction is usually associated with crampy abdominal pain, nausea, and sometimes vomiting. You may have increased diarrhea, or you may stop passing stool, and even gas, completely. Acute obstruction is not a complication of either Crohn's or ulcerative colitis.

If you have chronic obstruction, which is partial, you will experience abdominal pain, nausea, and bloating of the abdomen after meals. The interval between the meal and the symptoms depends on the site of blockage. Less than one hour suggests small bowel; more than one hour suggests colon.

Perforations, Abscesses, and Fistulas

Perforations can occur in both ulcerative colitis and Crohn's disease. Abscesses and fistulas are complications of Crohn's disease only.

Perforations are holes that develop in the wall of any hollow structure. As a result the bowel contents (including bacteria) leak into the abdominal cavity. If a perforation develops rapidly, the intestinal contents will spill into the peritoneal cavity and cause peritonitis. This is called a "free" perforation. The vast majority of free perforations in ulcerative colitis occur with toxic megacolon (see above). Free perforations can also occur in attacks of severe colitis without megacolon (i.e., toxic colitis), but such events are rare. Free perforations are also rare in Crohn's disease, except with toxic megacolon. The treatment in both ulcerative colitis and Crohn's disease is emergency surgery.

If a perforation develops slowly, the body usually reacts by "walling off" the hole in the bowel wall so that peritonitis does not result. This is called a "confined" perforation and results in the formation of an abscess (popularly called a "boil"). An abscess is a walled-off collection of pus. As explained earlier, pus is made up of a mixture of live and dead bacteria and live and dead white blood cells, with or without living and dead cells from adjacent tissues. An abscess can be virtually any size, from tiny and visible only under a microscope to something the size of a golfball, or larger.

A fistula, as we've seen, is an abnormal connection between

two hollow structures (such as bowel and bladder or bowel and vagina) or between a hollow structure and the skin. Once a fistula has been created, by the burrowing nature of the inflammation in Crohn's disease or by drainage (spontaneous or surgical) of an abscess, it is likely to drain intermittently or constantly. Antibiotics are often helpful. If the problem persists, surgery may be necessary.

Peri-anal Disease

Strictly speaking, this term refers to disease around the anus. But from a practical point of view it includes disease within the anal canal, as well as around it.

Hemorrhoids

Any condition that causes diarrhea or constipation is likely to lead to enlargement of the veins within the anal canal. The enlarged veins are known as hemorrhoids, or "piles." They are often felt as soft bumps protruding from the anal canal or immediately around it. Uncomplicated hemorrhoids don't hurt.

Occasionally a hemorrhoid becomes blocked by a blood clot. This is called a "thrombosed hemorrhoid." It causes considerable pain in the region of the anus, and the sufferer will likely be unwilling – or even unable – to sit. The pain is relieved dramatically if the hemorrhoid ruptures or if a surgeon makes a small cut in it to relieve the tension in the vein wall and surrounding tissues.

Skin Tags

When hemorrhoids bulge, they stretch the overlying skin. When the hemorrhoids shrink, the stretched skin remains and is commonly referred to as a "skin tag." In Crohn's disease, but not in ulcerative colitis, these tags can become swollen and firm. Once tags thicken, they usually stay that way. They don't hurt, but they are annoying to some patients, especially because bits of stool can get trapped between them and this can lead to chronic irritation of the skin and itching. In most people with Crohn's disease, it is best to avoid surgical removal of these swollen tags.

Anal Fissures

Many patients with hemorrhoids also develop anal fissures. An anal fissure is a cut or tear in the skin of the anal canal. This skin is extremely sensitive, so fissures can be quite painful, especially during a bowel movement and shortly after. The pain is often felt as a stretching or tearing during a bowel movement and as a burning afterward. Patients with Crohn's disease sometimes get fissures that are wider, longer, and deeper than those that occur in ulcerative colitis. When a fissure becomes deep, it becomes covered with a layer of pus and may be referred to as an "anal ulcer."

Abscesses and Fistulas

Many people with Crohn's disease develop abscesses and fistulas in and around the anus. A detailed discussion of how these develop and how they are treated appears in Chapter 7.

Strictures of the Anal Canal

These are common in Crohn's disease. If your stools are very loose, you will be unaware of the narrowing. When stools are formed, the diameter of the stool is restricted by the diameter of the stricture. People with strictures have narrow stools, but many people with narrow stools don't have strictures! The simple act of straining to have a bowel movement prevents the anal sphincter from relaxing properly, and this forces the stool to be squeezed out through a narrower passage.

Mild anal strictures need no treatment. More severe strictures may require periodic stretching. This can be done manually with the doctor's gloved finger or with instruments known as dilators.

Iron-Deficiency Anemia, Hemorrhage, and Massive Hemorrhage

"Anemia" means that the blood contains a reduced number of circulating red blood cells. It can be due to a deficiency of iron, folate (a B vitamin), or vitamin B_{12}. But even when these nutrients are present in adequate amounts, some people are anemic simply as a result of having a chronic disease. Chronic inflammation in the body suppresses the blood-producing activity of the bone marrow.

Folate deficiency can occur if you are taking sulfasalazine (see Chapter 6) or you are severely malnourished. Vitamin B_{12} deficiency may occur if you have extensive ileal disease, or after surgical removal of the ileum (see Chapter 7). Iron deficiency, however, is a little more complicated.

Anemia due to iron deficiency can develop in one of three ways. You may not be getting enough iron in your diet; this is uncommon in North America, but it is possible, especially if you eat little red meat or organ meats such as liver. Even if you have enough iron in your diet, you may not be absorbing it for some reason. And if you consume and absorb enough iron but still have iron deficiency, the only other possibility is that you are losing more iron than you are taking in. The way we lose iron is by losing blood. You can lose up to an ounce and a half (40 milliliters) of blood a day in the stool without seeing anything, if the bleeding comes from high enough up in the GI tract that the blood is thoroughly mixed in with the stool. Losing small amounts of blood on a daily basis will lead to iron-deficiency anemia over a period of several months.

Anemia in Ulcerative Colitis

No one with a recent onset of ulcerative colitis should have iron-deficiency anemia. Even though there is obviously blood in the stool, the amount is almost always less than you think; it takes very little bright red fluid to color a whole bowl of toilet water red! Unless bleeding is truly heavy, the bone marrow is able to use available stores of iron to keep the red-blood-cell count in the normal range. If you have had several attacks of ulcerative colitis, however, you will likely require some iron supplementation, since the stores of iron within the body eventually get used up.

Occasionally the bleeding is heavier than average and anemia may develop before the body has a chance to respond and produce new red blood cells.

Anemia in Crohn's Disease

Even in the absence of visible bleeding, people with Crohn's disease frequently develop iron-deficiency anemia. There are usually multiple ulcers (open sores) in the small or large intestine, and chronic, continuous, low-grade blood loss is common.

Sudden episodes of visible bleeding can occur, but not often. This happens when an ulcer burrows into a large blood vessel, generally a small artery. Fortunately, the normal repair mechanisms of the body usually seal off the bleeding vessel. In some people sudden bleeding of this type occurs only once, but in others it recurs or becomes persistent, and may require surgical treatment.

If people with extensive disease in the ileum or an extensive ileal resection are not given vitamin B_{12}, they may eventually develop anemia, because they may be less able to absorb vitamin B_{12} from food. The need for B_{12} can be determined with a Schilling test (see Chapter 7).

Massive Hemorrhage

Rarely in Crohn's disease, and very rarely in ulcerative colitis, sudden and massive bleeding occurs. In Crohn's disease, sudden massive bleeding may start in a patient who is otherwise feeling well, or during an attack. In most cases the source of such bleeding is the colon. Emergency surgery removes the colon. If the source of bleeding is the small intestine, the diseased segment will likely have to be removed. Even if bleeding stops spontaneously, the occurrence of a life-threatening hemorrhage usually necessitates removing the diseased bowel to avoid another, possibly fatal hemorrhage.

In ulcerative colitis, massive hemorrhage generally happens during a severe attack. Here the inflammatory process goes more deeply into the intestinal wall than usual and disrupts larger blood vessels. Surgical removal of the colon is often necessary.

Complications Outside the Intestine

Inflammatory bowel disease is associated with numerous complications outside the intestines. The areas commonly involved include the joints, the skin, the mouth, the liver, the bile duct, the kidneys, the blood, and the eyes.

Painful Joints

Ten to 20 percent of people with IBD have joint pains at some time. Joint disease associated with intestinal disease is referred to as *enteropathic arthropathy*. *Arthralgia* means joint pain. *Arthritis* refers to joints that are inflamed. A person with arthritis also has arthralgia, but many people with arthralgia do not have arthritis. I make this distinction because patients with joint pains often say that they have arthritis, but notice that their doctor does not use that term. From the patient's point of view, the terminology may not matter very much.

Arthritis associated with IBD is nondestructive: that is, the inflamed joints are not permanently damaged, as they are in rheumatoid or gouty arthritis, for example. You may have a lot of pain and swelling, but it is temporary, with no long-lasting effects.

Typically, arthritis of IBD occurs mainly in the large joints (e.g., knees, ankles) and tends to move from one joint to another. It may flare up when the IBD flares up, and settle down when the IBD settles down. However, it can precede any bowel symptoms by several years and can flare up when the bowel disease is relatively quiet. If the inflamed bowel is surgically removed, this form of arthritis goes away. Of course, if the disease is Crohn's disease and it recurs, then the arthritis may recur.

Ankylosing Spondylitis (AS or Sacroiliitis)

This is a type of arthritis involving the sacroiliac joints, with or without involvement of the joints of the spine. You may have pain or stiffness in the lower back, though such symptoms are more often due to ordinary spinal-disc disease. If the disease is looked for with X-rays and other tests, it is found in many people who do not have symptoms. As with arthritis, this condition can precede the onset of bowel symptoms by several years. Unlike arthritis, the symptoms of ankylosing spondylitis do not correlate at all with bowel disease activity, and do not improve after surgery on the bowel.

Ankylosing spondylitis can also occur independently of IBD, and is indistinguishable from AS in people with IBD. AS occurs in association with ulcerative colitis much more than with Crohn's disease.

Bone Disease

Osteonecrosis

This term literally means "bone death." It was previously

thought that osteonecrosis in patients with IBD was always a complication of steroid therapy. Recently, however, it was reported in two IBD patients who had never received steroids. The two most typical locations are the hips and the knees. This condition is extremely uncommon, but it can cause considerable disability. It leads to damage (known as avascular necrosis) of the hip or knee joints and usually requires artificial total hip or knee replacement.

Soft Bones

People with IBD frequently have osteoporosis. This is often blamed solely on steroid therapy, but is more likely related to a combination of factors, including low calcium intake, lack of exercise, steroid use, and possibly an inherited tendency to develop osteoporosis. In recent years, with the advent of a test known as bone densitometry, monitoring of bone health has become considerably more accurate. This test involves a minimal amount of radiation. It is brief (about 20 minutes), painless, and safe. Prior to this diagnostic technique, we had to rely on bone X-rays, which do not reveal evidence of osteoporosis until it is far advanced, or bone biopsy (removing a sample of bone), which is not practical for screening large numbers of patients.

Both calcium and vitamin D are necessary to form bone. As we saw in Chapter 5, vitamin D is available in food and vitamin supplements, and is also produced in the body when the skin is exposed to sunlight. People with Crohn's disease who have had more than a yard (about a meter) of ileum removed may not be able to absorb enough vitamin D and, possibly, calcium. They may be particularly susceptible to osteoporosis. The risk increases in postmenopausal female patients. In some patients, measuring blood levels of vitamin D is helpful. But vitamin D levels in some North Americans vary considerably with the seasons, because they are exposed to so much less sunlight during the winter months.

Sores in the Mouth

About 5 to 10 percent of people with IBD experience intermittent sores in the mouth. These are sometimes indistinguishable from the canker sores (also known as aphthous ulcers) that occur in the general population. However, canker sores in the general population generally occur one at a time, last a few days, and go away. Canker sores in IBD patients often occur in clusters, may be unusually large, and may persist for many days, even a few weeks. These sores usually occur when bowel disease is more active.

In addition to ordinary canker sores, people with Crohn's disease can develop mouth or throat ulcerations that look like Crohn's ulcers in the bowel. Biopsies of these ulcers show microscopic changes typical of Crohn's disease. There is no specific therapy available for this problem. Fortunately, these ulcers resolve themselves over a week or two in most patients.

Recent studies show that people with symptomatic Crohn's disease also have more gum infections and cavities than those whose disease is not causing any symptoms. This may simply

---

Treating Canker Sores in the Mouth

A treatment proven to be of some value in treating canker sores in the mouth is as follows. You need capsules (250 milligrams each) of the antibiotic tetracycline. Dissolve the contents of one capsule into one or two teaspoons (5 to 10 milliliters) of warm water. Hold the solution in your mouth for 10 to 15 minutes (if you can do it for that long!) and then spit it out. Try to do this four times a day. You should begin this treatment right at the onset of any fresh sores, and continue it for a few days. This can shorten the duration of the sores. Apply the local anesthetic viscous lidocaine directly onto the sores with a Q-Tip just before meals to decrease discomfort during eating.

be due to a difference in diet; some people with Crohn's disease eat an unusually large amount of refined sugars, to replace energy lost by avoidance of other foods.

Skin Diseases

The most common skin abnormality in IBD is *erythema nodosum*. It occurs in 2 to 10 percent of patients with IBD, and is somewhat more common in women. It consists of painful, tender red bumps that appear most often on the shins but sometimes show up on other parts of the legs, or even on the arms. It is often associated with a flare-up of IBD, and usually improves as the bowel disease is treated and improves.

Pyoderma gangrenosum (PG) occurs in 1 to 5 percent of people with IBD, and is more common in ulcerative colitis. Most people with PG have extensive colitis. PG begins with a raised, red, tender area of skin which then takes on the appearance of a blister. The roof of the blister breaks down and the result is a skin ulcer. PG usually occurs in multiple locations more or less simultaneously, and the ulcers can be any size, from tiny to extensive. Although these sores are generally painless, they are very unsightly and unpleasant to deal with, and some patients require extensive dressings.

Diseases of the Liver and Biliary Tract

Fatty liver

Fatty liver is a common complication in IBD. The cause is unknown, but in most cases it is likely malnutrition. Most patients have no symptoms or signs of the condition, it is not serious, and it is usually temporary.

Primary Sclerosing Cholangitis (PSC)

This is one of the most serious complications of IBD. It occurs in 1 to 4 percent of patients, more in patients with ulcerative colitis than in those with Crohn's disease. Some people with this condition do not have IBD, but about 70 percent do. "Primary" is a medical way of saying that the cause of the condition is unknown.

"Sclerosing" means "hardening." This disease causes scarring

Sclerosing Cholangitis

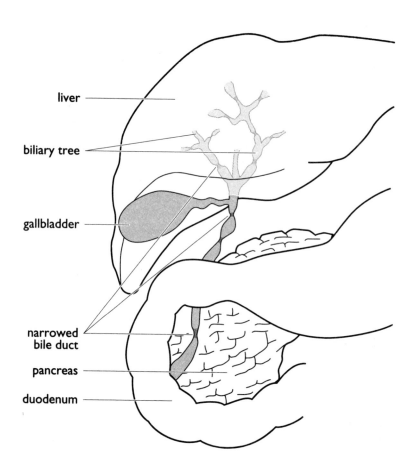

liver

biliary tree

gallbladder

narrowed bile duct

pancreas

duodenum

in the biliary tree along with inflammation of the bile duct and/or its branches. The scarring is patchy. It can be present only in the bile duct outside the liver, only in the branches of the biliary tree within the liver, or in both locations.

PSC is diagnosed by doing an ERCP – endoscopic retrograde cholangio-pancreatography – which involves injecting dye into the bile duct. Until the 1980s, no satisfactory treatment, medical or surgical, existed for PSC. Patients died of infection in the liver or of complications of liver damage that eventually results from untreated PSC. In the 1980s, cyclosporine was introduced to the field of transplantation. This drug alone was responsible for moving liver transplants from the back pages of newspapers to the front pages. Because of cyclosporine, the success rate in liver transplants increased from 20 percent to 80 percent or more.

Thus, since the mid-1980s, the treatment of choice for patients with *advanced* sclerosing cholangitis has been a liver transplant. Even so, patients with PSC still have a significantly reduced life expectancy compared with IBD patients without PSC, though it is considerably better than it used to be.

The development of new medications for the treatment of other liver and biliary-tract diseases has led to renewed interest in drug therapy for PSC. No drug has yet been proven to arrest or even slow its progression. Current studies are using a bile acid named "ursodeoxycholic acid" (referred to simply as "urso" or UDCA), alone or in combination with the immunosuppressive drug methotrexate (see Chapter 6).

Cancer of the Gall Bladder or Bile Ducts

Cancer of the gallbladder or bile ducts occurs in about 1 percent of patients with IBD, which is 10 to 20 times more often than these tumors occur in the general population. The tumors are more likely with ulcerative colitis than with Crohn's disease.

Gallstones

Bile salts are chemicals produced by the liver. They pass down from the liver into the duodenum dissolved in bile, and help to digest and absorb fat. Cholesterol is also dissolved in bile. Patients with extensive disease in the ileum or patients who have had some of the ileum surgically removed absorb and recycle a smaller percentage of the daily bile-salt output. Since one of the functions of bile salts is to keep the cholesterol in bile dissolved, the reduced level of bile salts allows more cholesterol to come out of solution and form stones in the gallbladder. This applies to patients with Crohn's disease only. At the present time, no effort is made to try to prevent these stones from developing. However, many gallstones never cause any symptoms and never require any treatment.

Kidney Stones

Kidney stones, usually composed of either calcium oxalate or uric acid, are much more common in people with IBD than they are in the general population. Most of the increased frequency is in people who have had surgery with removal of bowel.

How Can Kidney Stones Be Prevented?

As with many conditions, prevention is most desirable, if possible. If a patient who has had a resection of some kind has looser stools than normal, increasing oral fluid intake and reducing fluid loss in the stool is a good idea. Ileostomy patients are generally advised to consume at least two quarts (about two liters) of fluid a day. However, this is not always possible. Using an antidiarrheal drug such as loperamide or diphenoxylate (see Chapter 6) can be very effective in reducing fluid losses in the stool. Some physicians routinely prescribe low-oxalate diets for patients who have had an extensive ileal resection and/or those with extensive ileal disease, to reduce the risk of calcium oxalate stones.

What If Stones Are Already Present?

Most stones will pass through the urinary tract spontaneously. Stones stuck within a ureter often need to be treated by a urologist, a specialist in diseases of the urinary system. Stones that remain in the kidney are sometimes not treated but are monitored with ultrasound. The pain of kidney stones is not always typical. It is usually in the back, but sometimes it is felt in the abdomen, particularly below the waist on one side or the other. This may initially make you and your doctor think that the pain is due to the IBD. If the pain is not like your usual pain, consider the possibility of a kidney stone.

Hydronephrosis

This term literally means "water kidney." If a ureter is blocked, then the back-pressure on the kidney from the excess urine that cannot pass will cause the urine-collecting system to become stretched. If this persists, the pressure on the kidney can permanently damage it. Most cases occur in people with Crohn's ileitis, due to pressure on the lower end of the right ureter from the inflammatory process. Hydronephrosis is easily diagnosed with ultrasound, and mild cases may improve without surgery.

Amyloidosis

This rare disease causes widespread protein deposits in organs and tissues throughout the body. These deposits damage or destroy cells and interfere with organ function. Amyloidosis can occur in people who have no other disease, as well as in association with a variety of chronic diseases.

When it comes to IBD, amyloidosis occurs mainly with

Crohn's disease, and only rarely in patients with ulcerative colitis. It has been found in up to 25 percent of Crohn's patients studied at autopsy, but is found in only about 1 percent of living patients – and in many of these people, it is not causing any problems. However, when amyloidosis does cause serious illness, it is generally because it involves the kidneys, with kidney failure as an eventual result. Some experts think that amyloidosis can stabilize or even regress if the IBD is surgically removed, but some studies have shown no benefit at all. There has been limited success in treating this complication with colchicine, a medication that has been available for many, many years to treat acute gout. For patients in whom the progression of amyloidosis cannot be halted, dialysis and kidney transplantation remain possible alternatives.

Eye Problems

Eye disease, associated with either IBD or its treatment, occurs in about 10 percent of patients, though many cases are mild and are not brought to a doctor's attention. There are three main inflammatory conditions: conjunctivitis, episcleritis, and uveitis. Cataracts can occur as a complication of steroid therapy (see Chapter 6).

The occurrence of these inflammatory conditions may not correspond to how active the bowel disease is. Inflammation in the eye usually requires local treatment, which is often in the form of steroid drops.

Conjunctivitis (inflammation of the membrane lining and bordering the eyelids) is the most common condition, but it is not absolutely clear that this is a feature of IBD, since it is also common in the general population. Conjunctivitis can be unpleasant, but it is not serious.

Episcleritis (inflammation of the white of the eye) occurs in 3 to 4 percent of IBD patients, mostly those with Crohn's colitis. Patients usually complain of burning in one eye, and increased tear production. There may be some mild localized redness. This condition is also minor.

Uveitis (inflammation of the colored part of the eye), which occurs in 0.5 to 3 percent of patients, mainly in males with ulcerative colitis, can lead to serious loss of vision and requires treatment by an ophthalmologist. Patients with uveitis suddenly develop blurred vision, headaches, and eye pain. In rare patients, this problem can occur repeatedly. There is considerable controversy about how to treat this condition.

Blood-Clotting Abnormalities

It is well recognized that some IBD patients have abnormalities of the blood-clotting mechanism, resulting in an increased tendency to form blood clots in otherwise healthy blood vessels. There are approximately 13 different chemicals known as "clotting factors," some of which are increased in some patients with IBD. In addition, many patients have an elevated platelet count, especially during flare-ups of the bowel disease. Platelets are blood cells that are very important in the formation of blood clots.

Certain conditions predispose many sick patients, with a variety of acute and chronic diseases, to develop unwanted blood clots. Patients who are bedridden or dehydrated (whether it be due to fever, vomiting, diarrhea, or any other cause) are said to be in a "hypercoagulable" state, meaning that they are more prone to unwanted clots.

Most of the clots in IBD patients are in veins. The common locations are the leg veins and pelvic veins, but veins anywhere in the body can be involved.

To some extent, this problem can be circumvented if you

avoid prolonged periods of immobility. Patients who must stay in bed should be encouraged to wiggle their toes, bend their knees, and generally exercise their limbs. Isometric exercises are often very helpful. I always tell my patients that, when visitors come, it should not be just to talk. Visitors should be enlisted to help the patient exercise. Simple things like having the patient push each foot downward against the resistance of another person's hand can be very useful. You can easily make up similar exercises involving the use of other leg muscles or arm muscles. Patients not confined to bed should be encouraged to get out of bed, even if they don't feel like it.

In some situations doctors give bedridden patients low doses of anticoagulants ("blood thinners") to reduce the risk of unwanted blood clotting. The technology for doing this is quite advanced and poses little risk to the patient. If a patient does develop a clot, the usual treatment is an anticoagulant.

Pancreatitis

Inflammatory disease of the pancreas has occasionally been reported in association with IBD for many years. Many of the cases are clearly due to taking certain medications: sulfasalazine, 5-aminosalicylate, azathioprine, and 6-mercaptopurine (see Chapter 6). Other cases link pancreatitis with Crohn's disease but not ulcerative colitis.

Cancer Complicating IBD

Patients with either ulcerative colitis or Crohn's colitis have more risk of cancer of the colon than the general population, and patients with small-bowel Crohn's disease have an increased risk of cancer of the small bowel. Detailed information on this topic is found in Chapter 10.

Nutritional Complications of IBD

Malnutrition – characterized by low body weight, sometimes with vitamin or mineral deficiencies – is a common problem. See Chapter 5 for details.

TEN

Cancer and IBD

U p till the end of the 1950s, people with ulcerative colitis, but not those with Crohn's disease, were thought to have an increased risk of colon cancer. At that time, Crohn's disease was felt to involve only the small intestine, and all colitis was felt to be ulcerative colitis. At the end of the 1950s and the beginning of the 1960s, however, medical researchers in Britain and North America concluded that Crohn's disease could occur in the colon, though it was uncommon. Now we know that Crohn's disease not only occurs in the colon, but is common there.

Before 1970 many colon-cancer patients who were said to have ulcerative colitis actually had Crohn's disease of the colon. It is now generally accepted that the cancer risk in Crohn's colitis is probably the same as the cancer risk for ulcerative colitis. People with small-bowel Crohn's disease also have an increased risk of small-bowel cancer. However, cancer of the small intestine is extremely rare in the general population. Even with the increased risk associated with Crohn's disease, it is still a very uncommon event.

Who Is at Risk?

Ulcerative Colitis

Two factors determine the risk of cancer in patients with ulcerative colitis: how much of the colon is (or has been) inflamed, and the total duration of the disease.

Generally speaking, the more colon involved, the greater the risk. Patients who have proctitis (colitis limited to the rectum) have a risk equal to that of the general population. Over the past several years we've learned that colon cancer is at least partly genetically determined. There are therefore two groups in the "general population": those with no family history of colon polyps (the forerunners of most colon cancers) or colon cancer; and those with a family history of colon polyps and/or cancer. We still don't know what effect family history has on the colon-cancer risk in ulcerative colitis patients.

The risk of cancer is also thought to increase with every year that passes from the time the disease began. During the first ten years of disease this risk is just fractionally above that of the general population. After ten years, the risk is more substantial. Actual numbers aren't given because there is such wide variation in the medical literature.

Crohn's Disease

The age of the patient at the time Crohn's disease first began is felt to be the most important factor in determining cancer risk in people with Crohn's colitis. Patients diagnosed prior to age 20 are at the greatest risk. However, the magnitude of the risk is uncertain. The extent and duration of the disease (independent of age at onset) may also be factors in colon-cancer risk, but these are not as well established as in ulcerative colitis.

As for cancer of the small bowel in patients with small-bowel Crohn's disease, we still don't know the factors that influence the risk, with one exception.

Up to about 25 years ago, an operation known as "exclusion bypass" – the diseased ileum was not removed, but the normal ileum upstream was disconnected and reconnected to the colon – was performed on some patients with small-bowel Crohn's disease. This operation is no longer done, but there are still many people who have had the surgery. There have been several reports of patients developing cancer in the piece of excluded ileum. Because the flow of intestinal contents is diverted and does not pass through this part of the ileum, symptoms and signs of this cancer usually appear late and the area is difficult to investigate with a scope or barium enema. It is now felt that if a patient who previously had an exclusion bypass is having abdominal surgery for any reason, the excluded section of ileum should be removed to eliminate any chance of cancer in this area.

Reducing the Risk

In the late 1970s and all through the 1980s, colonoscopy became more and more commonplace and easier and easier to do. It seemed obvious that examining the colon at regular intervals would lead to earlier cancer detection. Also in the late 1970s, two British pathologists named Morson and Pang described a microscopic change referred to as *dysplasia* (a change in cell architecture) in the colon biopsies of patients with colitis and early cancer. A progression from mild dysplasia to severe dysplasia to cancer was found, and was thought to have some value in predicting which patients were likely to go on to get colon cancer. Now we know that if the colon is completely removed in patients with severe dysplasia, about half of them will turn out to have cancer; it can be detected by the pathologist, even though the tumor was not visible through the endoscope.

Nevertheless, surveillance testing is extremely controversial. In this age of concern about healthcare costs, it is not at all clear that surveillance colonoscopy is "cost effective" in patients with chronic colitis, be it ulcerative or Crohn's. Some studies show a relative inability to detect precancerous disease either with the endoscope or under the microscope. Other studies report that regular surveillance colonoscopy has led to the early diagnosis of cancer or even precancer.

How Often Should Surveillance Colonoscopy Be Done?

Just as there is no agreement about whether surveillance colonoscopy should be done at all, there is no agreement about how often it should be done. Some gastroenterologists do the procedure once a year. Others do it once every two years. Still others do a full colonoscopy every two years, with a flexible sigmoidoscopy in the years in between. Patients with total colitis often have significant shortening of their colon, and flexible sigmoidoscopy has a good chance of screening at least the lower half (left side plus part of transverse) of the colon. There is some evidence that a patient who has cancer or severe dysplasia on the right side of the colon will also have dysplasia on the left side.

If a patient has less than half the colon affected by colitis, most gastroenterologists will do surveillance examinations less frequently. There is no question that a cancer risk still exists for people with involvement of a third to half of the colon, but the risk is smaller and the enthusiasm of both the patient and the doctor is understandably less. Nevertheless, some gastroenterologists still examine the colon every year. If the colitis is clearly confined to the rectum and sigmoid, some gastroenterologists don't do surveillance at all; others do. Only when the disease is clearly confined to the rectum is there general agreement that surveillance colonoscopy is not necessary.

How Often Should a Surveillance Exam for Cancer be Performed?

Ulcerative colitis: Not all specialists agree. At present, some advise a colonoscopy yearly, some advise one every two years, and some advise a surveillance colonoscopy every two years with a flexible sigmoidoscopy in the years in between.

Crohn's colitis: People with Crohn's colitis should probably have surveillance just as frequently as people with ulcerative colitis. But this has been decided only recently, and not all gastroenterologists feel surveillance is needed. Many patients with Crohn's disease of the colon have never been advised to have a surveillance colonoscopy. If you are such a patient, discuss this with your doctor.

Crohn's disease of the small intestine: There is no practical method of inspecting the small bowel. You must rely on the experience and judgment of your doctor. Symptoms that are atypical for you, or show a change in the pattern of your disease, should make you and your doctor give at least a passing thought to the possibility of cancer. But because cancer in small-bowel Crohn's disease is rare, most times the answer will lie elsewhere.

What about People with Small-Bowel Crohn's Disease?
There is no equivalent surveillance procedure for patients with small-bowel Crohn's disease. Enteroscopy (endoscopic examination of the small intestine) is impractical, and is restricted to certain patients. Some gastroenterologists X-ray the small bowel once every few years even if you are well, but the chance of picking up an asymptomatic cancer in this way is tiny.

Fortunately, small-bowel cancer, even in patients with Crohn's disease, is very uncommon.

ELEVEN

Living with IBD

The theme of the nineties is empowerment. In medicine, knowledge is the key to empowerment. The previous chapters have provided you with general information about your problem. This one focuses on more personal issues and suggests ways for dealing with these.

Sex and IBD

As with virtually any chronic disease, the patient with IBD is concerned about three main aspects of sex: sexual activity; fertility; contraception.

Sexual Activity

Understandably, a disease that has symptoms of abdominal pain and urgent and frequent bowel movements, and difficulty getting to the bathroom on time, can lead to decreased interest in sexual intercourse for both men and women.

Unfortunately, both doctors and patients tend to avoid talking about sexual activity. However, if a chronic problem is interfering with a sexual relationship, the issue should be considered important enough to warrant discussion and perhaps a change in therapy.

The Impact of Surgery on Sexual Activity

As a result of improved general health after diseased bowel is removed, surgery generally brings an increased libido and improved sexual relationships. However, certain types of surgery clearly produce psychological difficulties.

Most people adapt well to a standard Brooke ileostomy and appliance (see Chapter 7), but concern over body image can result in great anxiety, which in turn can interfere significantly with sexual activity. This is especially true in young singles.

One of the most distressing things that can happen to a patient with a Brooke ileostomy is that the appliance can suddenly become dislodged, or can leak during sexual intercourse. Coping with this requires maturity and a "grin and bear it" attitude. Understandably, if this happens even once, the fear that it will happen again is strongly inhibiting. Fortunately, ileostomy appliances have improved significantly over the years, and such events are uncommon.

Patients with a properly functioning Kock (continent) ileostomy are usually not troubled by leaking stool. However, men undergoing total colectomy to establish a continent ileostomy have approximately a 2 percent risk of impotence. This is because the nerves that control erection are in the same vicinity as those to the anus and rectum; nerve damage during surgery can be a complication.

Women undergoing total colectomy frequently develop increased vaginal fluid production without signs of infection. In many of these patients, this results in a rather heavy vaginal discharge that is annoying, at least. About one in four women having a total colectomy complains of painful sexual intercourse – twice as many as the number of women with this complaint before such surgery. Similarly, men may complain of reduced libido and sexual satisfaction after such surgery. However, despite these problems, the majority of total-colectomy patients report an overall improvement in their sex life.

Men undergoing a near-total colectomy with pelvic-pouch procedure and ileo-anal anastomosis have a 1 to 2 percent risk of impotence. There is also a 3 to 4 percent risk of retrograde ejaculation (see Chapter 7). Because this type of surgery is often associated with mild diarrhea and episodes of incontinence, both men and women may feel anxious during sexual intercourse. Nevertheless, as with other types of surgery, sexual life generally improves overall, likely due to better general health.

Fertility

Most studies of patients with ulcerative colitis have shown no evidence of impaired fertility in either men or women. Not so for Crohn's disease. Women with *active* Crohn's disease are somewhat less likely to become pregnant and men with *active* Crohn's disease who are in ill health or undernourished may have difficulty fathering a child.

We don't know what causes reduced fertility in women with Crohn's disease. It may be that the bowel disease somehow creates blockages of the fallopian tubes. However, fertility may actually be normal, and the reduced number of pregnancies may be a result of either medical advice to avoid pregnancy or such severe pain on intercourse that it is avoided.

There is some evidence that patients with Crohn's disease who are treated surgically may have higher fertility than those who are treated with drugs and/or diet therapy. Presumably this relates to improved general health. If general health improved sufficiently without surgery, the same improvement might be seen.

Sulfasalazine (see Chapter 6) can reduce the sperm count enough to result in male infertility. Fortunately this abnormality is reversible, though it takes two to three months for the sperm count to return to normal after the drug is stopped. None of the other medications commonly used for IBD is known to interfere with fertility.

Contraception

All forms of contraception can be used by patients with IBD.

There is no evidence that the birth control pill interacts with any of the medications used to treat IBD, but there is some evidence that it may aggravate the symptoms of some women with Crohn's disease. However, this is controversial and is certainly not a reason to avoid the pill. If you are on the pill and you are wondering if you should stop it, discuss this with your gastroenterologist.

The Menstrual Cycle and IBD

Recent studies have shown that women with irritable bowel syndrome (see Chapter 4) are likely to experience an increase in their symptoms just before and during menstrual periods. Similarly, many women with IBD complain that their symptoms become worse when they get their period. But this has not been well studied to date, and strategies to help patients deal with the problem have not yet been designed.

Pregnancy and IBD

Here are some commonly asked questions, and some answers.

What Effect Can My IBD Have on a Pregnancy?

Ulcerative colitis and Crohn's disease generally do not have any adverse effects on pregnancy. Most babies are normal and full-term. Deliveries are no more complicated than usual and there is no increase in the need for forceps or caesarian sections.

If the disease is active *before* conception, the risks of a miscarriage or premature birth are slightly increased, more so in

Crohn's disease than in ulcerative colitis. If a severe attack of IBD occurs *during* a pregnancy, the chances for a normal delivery and a healthy baby are slightly reduced. If the symptoms of ulcerative colitis *first* occur during a pregnancy, the chances for a normal delivery and a healthy baby are very good.

Crohn's disease that appears for the first time during pregnancy may have a poorer outcome. However, in comparison with ulcerative colitis, there have been relatively few reports of Crohn's disease beginning during pregnancy. When it has been reported, there has been a significantly higher rate of fetal death. This information applies *only* to Crohn's disease that appears for the *first* time during pregnancy.

Does Pregnancy Increase the Risk of a Flare-up of IBD?

For anyone in remission, there is a 30 percent chance of a relapse during the next year. Pregnancy neither increases nor reduces that chance. If a flare-up does occur around this time, it will more likely happen in the first three months of pregnancy or soon after delivery. The behavior of the disease during one pregnancy cannot be used to predict what will happen in another pregnancy in the same woman.

Patients with Crohn's disease who have had surgery for Crohn's reportedly do much better during pregnancy than those who have never had surgery.

If My IBD Is Active When I Become Pregnant, What Effect Will the Pregnancy Have on the Disease?

If your disease is active at the time of conception, generally it will continue to be active during pregnancy. As when you are not pregnant, therapy should be aimed at controlling the disease.

Can Pregnancy Affect the Course of My IBD?

A recent study has suggested that women with Crohn's and a

previous pregnancy need surgery to remove diseased areas less often than those who have never been pregnant.

What about Abortion and IBD?

If pregnancy occurs while a woman is on the antibiotic metronidazole or on one of the immunosuppressive drugs (see Chapter 6), a therapeutic abortion is justifiable. In rare instances, a pregnancy may be terminated in a woman with severe active IBD. There is no evidence that therapeutic abortions carry any greater risks for women who have IBD than for those who don't.

Does an IBD Patient Need a Special Diet during Pregnancy?

Generally speaking, the normal, well-balanced diet that any pregnant woman should follow is fine. If your disease is active, however, you may have to pay extra attention to your diet. The most important thing is to make sure you are taking in enough energy for the fetus to develop and grow normally. Failure to gain weight at the expected rate is a sign that more energy is needed. Inflammation uses up energy, so extra intake may be necessary. Pregnant patients can be adequately nourished with enteral diets or total parenteral nutrition (see Chapter 5) if necessary.

Can I Take My IBD Drugs When I'm Pregnant?

Like anyone else, IBD patients should try to avoid *unnecessary* drugs during pregnancy. Fortunately, both sulfasalazine and steroids have proven safe for the fetus. There is no increased risk of prematurity, stillbirth, fetal deformity, or other congenital abnormalities. There is no increased danger of a full-term infant becoming jaundiced if you take sulfasalazine to the end of your pregnancy. But be sure to notify your pediatrician if you are on sulfasalazine, steroids, or narcotic medications.

It's very likely that 5-ASA will prove safe in pregnancy, but we don't know yet. Because 5-ASA is a component of sulfasalazine, and sulfasalazine, as we've said, is safe in pregnancy, there is every reason to believe that 5-ASA is also safe. Some preliminary reports have attested to the safety of this agent, but the reports are based on small numbers.

Immunosuppressive medications such as azathioprine and 6-mercaptopurine are generally *not* recommended during pregnancy. In fact, methotrexate has even been used (in large doses) to produce a therapeutic abortion. However, uneventful pregnancies have occurred in women taking these medications, and healthy babies have been born. Nevertheless, if conception occurs while a women is on one of these drugs, a therapeutic abortion may be medically indicated. The same is true for the antibiotics metronidazole and ciprofloxacin.

We don't have information about the safety of diphenoxylate and loperamide in pregnancy because no studies have been done. Codeine, the main alternative to these drugs, *has* been studied, and is associated with a very slight increase in risk to the fetus.

Can I Breastfeed My Baby?

If your disease is active at the time of delivery, you may not be able to provide sufficient milk. Sulfasalazine and 5-ASA do make their way into breast milk, but they present no hazard to the full-term infant if you are able to breastfeed. In rare cases the breastfed infant has had diarrhea because the mother was taking 5-ASA (tablets, enemas, or suppositories).

Steroids and antidiarrheal drugs also make their way into breast milk, and may cause side effects in infants. The risk is directly related to the dose. If you want to nurse your baby while you are on any of these drugs, the baby should be carefully monitored by a pediatrician. No information is available on the safety of loperamide during breastfeeding.

You should not breastfeed if you are on immunosuppressive drugs or the antibiotics metronidazole or ciprofloxacin.

Life Expectancy

Over the past 25 years, the life expectancy of patients with IBD has approached that of the general population. This is attributable to several factors, including earlier diagnosis, a greater range of therapies, better attention to nutrition, better surgical techniques, and much better care following surgery.

From a statistical point of view, the first attack of colitis (either type) is often the worst attack that the patient will experience. The risk of dying from an attack of acute colitis has become extremely low. In fact, the only measurable risk is associated with first attacks.

Ulcerative Colitis

Among the patients who initially have ulcerative proctitis, between 10 and 20 percent can expect to progress to more involvement of the colon, usually within the first 2 years but occasionally even after that. Among patients having ulcerative colitis involving the rectum and sigmoid colon, up to 50 percent may progress to more involvement of the colon, usually during the first 10 years of disease. The percentage of patients dying from ulcerative colitis has steadily declined over the past 20 years; the risk is greater than that of the general population only with the first attack. The lifetime risk of requiring colectomy is about 30 percent. However, more people with extensive colitis will need surgery than those with limited disease.

Crohn's Disease

Studies over the years have consistently shown a higher mortality risk in Crohn's disease than in ulcerative colitis. However, just as the risk of dying from ulcerative colitis has decreased greatly in the past 20 years, the same is true for Crohn's disease. It is currently thought that the mortality risk is close to, if not identical with, that of the general population. If there is an increase of mortality at all, it is in patients whose disease begins at a young age. Part of the increased risk of dying in this group appears to be related to the development of cancer.

In the long term, patients with Crohn's disease can expect surgery much more often than patients with ulcerative colitis. Taking patients with all forms of Crohn's disease, the probability of requiring some kind of surgery is about 80 percent. The average number of operations per patient in this group is approximately three. But these statistics include minor operations, such as draining a peri-anal abscess. Patients with small-bowel Crohn's disease who have had more than a yard (about a meter) of ileum removed are much more likely to have gallbladder stones and/or kidney stones compared with the general population, and compared with patients with Crohn's disease who have not had this extent of surgery.

Quality of Life with IBD

"Quality of life" has become an important measuring-stick for evaluating the effects of chronic diseases, and of various treatments. In the 1980s a group at McMaster University in Hamilton, Ontario, developed a quality-of-life index to evaluate patients with inflammatory bowel disease. This index has been used in a variety of studies, both nationally and internationally.

The index has proved to be extremely useful in assessing quality of life for patients with IBD. The index is not all-inclusive – items related to sexual activity and satisfaction are noteworthy by their absence. Nevertheless, studies have shown that the index score before and after medical or surgical treatment provides a relatively accurate assessment of the benefit, or lack of benefit, to the patient.

Quality-of-Life Index

This index evaluates quality of life according to five factors:

1. *Bowel symptoms*
   a) frequent bowel movements
   b) loose bowel movements
   c) abdominal cramps
   d) pain in the abdomen
   e) abdominal bloating
   f) passing large amounts of gas

2. *Systemic symptoms*
   a) fatigue
   b) overall feeling unwell
   c) feeling worn out
   d) tiring very easily
   e) waking up during the night
   f) feeling weak

3. *Emotional function*
   a) frustrated
   b) depressed
   c) discouraged
   d) fearful of not finding a washroom in time
   e) worried about surgery
   f) worried about flare-up
   g) irritable
   h) angry
   i) anxious
   j) impatient

4. *Social impairment*
   a) avoiding events where washrooms are not close at hand
   b) canceling social engagements
   c) being unable to play sports
   d) being unable to plan outings in advance

5. *Functional impairment*
   a) being unable to attend work/school regularly
   b) having to stop work/school
   c) having difficulty doing housework

Statistics can be very helpful, but in the end it comes down to each individual. A drug or surgical procedure that benefits most patients may not be looked on favorably by a given person. Furthermore, in studying any treatment choice, measuring the quality-of-life index *over a period of time* is desirable.

Let's take someone who has been continuously ill with Crohn's disease for several months. She is chronically fatigued, eating poorly, and taking multiple medications. Surgery is advised and performed. One month following surgery, she is feeling much better, is off almost all medications, and is eating well, and her quality of life is clearly much improved. She does have diarrhea, which is a result of the surgery, but she has been told that this is usually temporary and so she is optimistic.

Six months later the diarrhea has not gotten any better and the patient is now being told that this diarrhea – a result of surgery, not of Crohn's disease – is likely to be permanent, and that medication will be necessary to keep it under control. A quality-of-life measurement taken at this point is not as good. Three months later, the patient develops symptoms indicating that the Crohn's disease has recurred. Over the next few weeks she does poorly, develops an abscess, and is told that another operation will be necessary. At this point her quality of life is greatly colored by what has happened and what is going to happen, and the score is significantly reduced.

After the second operation, the patient is pessimistic. But as it turns out, there is no evidence of recurring Crohn's disease for the next five years. As the patient acclimatizes to chronic diarrhea requiring antidiarrheal therapy, her quality-of-life score steadily improves.

Other Factors Affecting Quality of Life

Losses

Developing a chronic disease may mean certain losses for the sufferer. If the disease is mild, losses will be minimal. However, if you are frequently or continuously ill the effects on life in general are likely to be significant. Unfortunately, personal relationships frequently suffer. It is not unusual for a healthy spouse to be unable to cope with chronic illness in a partner. Unmarried patients generally find it more difficult to establish lasting relationships. They may be embarrassed about the disease, or unable to participate in various activities because of restrictions the disease places on them, or may lack sufficient energy to engage in certain activities with a potential partner.

Having a chronic illness sometimes means a loss of independence. Patients who are frequently ill, especially if the illness requires hospitalization, need to depend on someone else to deal with such simple things as paying bills. One of the hardest things for most patients to accept is at least intermittent loss of the ability to control their own lives.

Anger

When older people develop a chronic illness, they may be upset, but they tend to accept it more easily than young people. As people get older, they see family and friends developing illnesses and expect to have some sort of problem sooner or later. Conversely, young people generally assume that everyone else in their age group is healthy, and their feeling is "Why me?" Of course, it's not true that all young people are well. Many young people have friends who have severe asthma and end up in emergency departments on a regular basis. Others have friends with severe diabetes who must inject insulin every day.

Still others have friends who have leukemia or some other form of cancer. Nevertheless it is true that most young people are healthy, and certainly the image of youth is constantly linked with the idea of health and energy in our culture.

Particularly in the initial stages of disease, the patient is likely to feel anger toward family, friends, and healthcare workers, all of whom are trying to be helpful but cannot know exactly how that person feels. Even when they are coping well, some patients are angry and frequently feel that "people don't understand." This may apply, in the patient's mind, to parents, teachers, co-workers, relatives, and friends. To some extent, this perception of a lack of understanding is true. Even if teachers or co-workers are told the name of the disease (and patients don't always want to advertise their problems), many people have no good understanding of what effects such diseases have on a person's life.

Especially when IBD is resistant to treatment, patients feel that days are like weeks and weeks are like months or years. They often temporarily lose confidence in their ability to overcome an attack of the illness. This pessimistic attitude and frustration with the disease may lead them to ignore treatment instructions, or at least to be careless about them.

Coping Strategies

If you have a chronic illness such as Crohn's disease or ulcerative colitis, there are many ways you can improve your situation and develop a more positive outlook.

First, accept the fact that you have the disease. Then try to learn about it. Learn about the treatments. Think of yourself and your healthcare providers as a team. Help them to help you; in this way you will help yourself. As has been said many times in relation to many other problems, take one day at a time.

When you feel well, eat well. Consider that a little extra weight is like money in the bank. Unless you are clearly over-weight, don't worry about gaining a few extra pounds. When your disease flares up and you lose weight, you will not be as badly off.

When you are in the hospital, try not to think of it as a prison. Get permission to go outside, weather permitting. Having an IV line, including a central line, does not mean you have to stay indoors. Even patients with various drainage tubes, drainage bags, bladder catheters, and other devices can go out. If you are on a tube feeding, don't be embarrassed and hide in your room. Getting out into fresh air (even polluted air!) improves outlook. Whether you are roaming the halls of the hospital or strolling outside, remind yourself that exercise is good for you. The more you strengthen your muscles, the more rapidly you will recover from the illness or operation that has led to your hospitalization.

If you are weak, the philosophy should be that *any* activity is better than no activity. I tell patients who are very weak to start by just sitting on the edge of the bed. The next step is to stand beside the bed, and after that to get out on one side of the bed, walk around the bed, and get in on the other side. I have had patients start out with limited activity such as this and end up literally running up and down the stairs of the hospital – carrying an IV pole! Being active has psychological rewards as well as physical ones. And there are other things you can do for yourself in hospital to make it feel more like home. Have family or friends bring your schoolwork, office work, or other work. If you have a portable computer (insured!), have them bring it in. Wear your own clothes, use your own pillow, and have someone bring you soft toilet paper!

If you know that antidiarrheal drugs effectively control your diarrhea or the urgency to go the bathroom, use them to give you psychological security when you are going out, whether to the theater, a sports event, a party, or simply the grocery store. Similarly, such medications can be helpful in sexual activity.

Be self-reliant. Learn which kinds of medical decisions you can make on your own. Don't feel that you have to ask your doctor everything. This will build your self-confidence and help to make you feel better.

Financial Effects of Chronic Disease

Perhaps one of the most difficult areas in maintaining quality of life is the financial burden of chronic disease. Government health plans may cover hospital costs and a few outpatient expenses, but some people do not have drug plans, and other people have drug plans that cover only part of the cost of medications, many of which are quite expensive. Disability insurance that adequately replaces a person's income is extremely expensive and inaccessible to many patients. Some pharmaceutical companies recognize these financial difficulties and provide free medication to the patient via the physician. However, during difficult economic times, when many individuals cannot afford the cost of medications, the demand greatly exceeds the supply. Not only does illness interfere with income, it also frequently makes it impossible to put any money away for retirement. This can obviously have far-reaching consequences on patients and their families.

Social Effects

A Danish study reviewed familial, social, and professional data on a group of patients with ulcerative colitis in comparison with a control group of patients of similar age and sex who were in hospital for a variety of acute illnesses. A higher percentage of colitis patients had university degrees, and fewer were unskilled workers. Patients had generally kept the same job for equal lengths of time in both groups. The colitis patients had the same frequency of marriage as the controls and seemed to have no more familial or sexual problems. The authors of this study constructed a score to rate social life. They included such items as frequency of visiting friends, and participating in cultural events, sports events, etc. About a third of the patients in both groups had very active social lives and about half had moderately active social lives; no differences were found between the ulcerative colitis patients and the controls. Similarly, a score was devised for physical activity, and again no difference was found. The authors concluded that patients with ulcerative colitis, despite their often troublesome disease, can lead normal lives, provided that they have access to appropriate medical and surgical care when they are ill.

Statistics related to family and social life are not as readily available for Crohn's disease. However, the overall quality of life is not as good, *on average*, for Crohn's patients as for ulcerative colitis patients. But of course both diseases appear in a wide spectrum, from something that is a minor nuisance to something that is a cause of major ongoing disability.

Parents and Children, Children and Parents

Most parents can adjust to chronic disease in themselves, and most children can do the same. However, when parents have to adjust to chronic illness in their children, there is sometimes an extreme tendency to be overprotective. At the same time the sick child goes into denial of illness, and becomes quite resistant to parental intervention.

Parents must try to allow the patient to develop a relationship with the doctor, particularly when the patient is a teenager or a young adult. Parents must give their children a chance to manage their disease independently, in the same way that they must learn to "let go" as healthy children grow up. By the same token, children should recognize that their parents genuinely care and are trying to help.

Parents – trust your kids! Be there to help them when they want help. Kids – respect your parents! If you want independence, show that you can be responsible. Take your medications without having to be reminded. Tell your doctor (and your parents) when you are sick. Keep your appointments.

Quality of life is, to a large extent, a personal perception. It reflects the way that a particular individual feels about his or her state of health as well as various other aspects of life in general. Many people expect to feel good all the time. Patients with IBD learn to recognize that this isn't possible. Accepting that there are going to be some "down times" is an important step in developing the ability to cope successfully with IBD. Patients who can learn self-reliance will be less tied to their doctors, and this will give them self-confidence and higher self-esteem.

Travel Tips

If you have taken the time to learn about your disease and its treatments, and to learn which medications you can start or adjust on your own and when you should use these medications, you should feel confident about traveling. Remember, many countries have IBD societies or foundations, and their members will be only too happy to help you get appropriate care should you need it. Many European countries have at least one hospital with English-speaking staff. Because IBD occurs worldwide, there are physicians and surgeons familiar with the condition worldwide.

The fact is, many knowledgeable IBD patients are aware that they can deal with most problems on their own. Sometimes all it takes is a telephone call to your gastroenterologist back home, for a little advice or to act as a "sounding board."

Don't forget your drugs, and take adequate supplies in your carry-on luggage. If you start to experience symptoms, act promptly. Patients frequently wait to see if a problem will just "settle down on its own." Generally speaking, this is not a good idea when you are away from home.

If you have ulcerative colitis and you begin to have a flare-up, you can increase your oral 5-ASA, start 5-ASA suppositories or enemas, or start hydrocortisone foam or liquid steroid enemas. If you are familiar with the use of steroids and think they are necessary, you can start taking them, provided your symptoms are typical and not dramatic. *If you think you are having a severe attack of colitis, seek medical advice locally.* High fever, vomiting, severe abdominal pain, and heavy bleeding are all signs of a potentially severe attack. If you treat yourself for a flare-up of colitis and then become very constipated, you can get your bowels moving again by using mineral oil or one of the other remedies described in Chapter 6.

If you have small-bowel Crohn's disease and think you are developing an obstruction, promptly put yourself on clear fluids. Keep them up for 36 to 48 hours, then gradually begin eating again, but leave roughage out of your diet for a few additional days. If you are on steroids, you should usually double the dose for a few days. You can go back to your previous dose if you settle down quickly, or taper back to your usual dose if you settle down slowly. If you are not on steroids, you will likely get over an obstruction just as fast without starting them. *If your pain is worse than usual, different from usual, or more persistent than usual, seek prompt medical assistance.*

If you have Crohn's disease and you develop symptoms of a flare-up without symptoms of obstruction, you are still likely to benefit by going on clear fluids for 36 to 48 hours. Many patients with Crohn's disease feel better if they don't eat. Just resting the bowel for a few days may be sufficient treatment. If the symptoms subside but promptly begin again when you start eating, you will clearly need medication, possibly steroids. Again, many knowledgeable patients start steroids on their own in this situation. If you are on a maintenance dose of a 5-ASA product, doubling the dose may be helpful, with steroid use as a "fall-back" position. Once again, *if the flare-up is different from usual or more severe than usual, seek medical help promptly.*

If you know what's happening, it is reasonable to try to treat yourself. If you can afford to go on a trip, you should be able to afford a telephone call to your gastroenterologist for a bit of advice or reassurance. If you don't know what's happening or you are not sure, it is foolish to take chances. In this situation, seek prompt medical assistance. If you feel it would be useful for the local doctor to speak to your gastroenterologist, you can request this and offer to pay for the communication, be it a phone call or a fax.

Employers and IBD

Crohn's disease, and to a lesser extent ulcerative colitis, has always had a bad reputation in the business world. Many employers are reluctant to hire people with IBD, although this discrimination is illegal. The perception is that the IBD patient will be ill frequently and will miss work. In fact, this may never happen. Patients and their doctors have become so good at dealing with most IBD problems on an outpatient basis that many people can keep working when they are ill, with the loss of very few days, if any.

In many ways, IBD patients are ideal employees. Most become toughened by the illness and are more likely to come to work when suffering relatively minor illnesses which would keep many otherwise healthy people at home. IBD patients are conscious of the risk of a flare-up and of having to miss significant periods of work. As a result, they try not to miss work for any other reason.

Studies have been done to examine discrimination against people with Crohn's disease in both school and the workplace. In one study, students with Crohn's lost significantly more days of school than healthy students but were as successful academically, as measured by the courses they completed and whether they entered university. Although discrimination against a potential employee on the basis of an illness is illegal, many Crohn's patients feel that they have been rejected for this reason, even though another excuse may have been given. As a result of such experiences, up to 30 percent of Crohn's patients conceal their illness from employers.

Insurance and IBD

For many years patients and their physicians have known that IBD is used as a reason to refuse insurance or to charge a high premium. A group of Canadian gastroenterologists recently undertook a study of the insurance industry's attitude to patients with IBD, and also looked at the issue from the patients' point of view.

The perception in the insurance industry was that patients with IBD might have some difficulty, but not a great deal of difficulty, in obtaining life insurance.

Not surprisingly, patients had a different opinion, based on their experiences. Of patients with Crohn's disease who applied for straight life insurance, only 18 percent were accepted without an extra premium; 44 percent were asked to pay extra, and 38 percent were rejected. For the same kind of insurance, the comparable figures for patients with ulcerative colitis were 31 percent, 36 percent, and 33 percent. The authors of the study believed that some patients likely do not even bother to apply for life insurance, because they are so certain they won't get it. This is probably true.

People with Crohn's disease applying for group insurance did surprisingly well – 83 percent were accepted. In comparison, only 65 percent of patients with ulcerative colitis said they had been accepted. Among those surveyed, only a small number of patients with Crohn's disease had applied for individual disability insurance. Of those, 41 percent were approved at standard rates and 23 percent had to pay an additional premium. In the ulcerative colitis group, a greater number of patients applied and 38 percent were rejected. Most patients who applied for group disability were accepted, but the number who applied was fairly low.

The study also looked at drug plans. For individual plans, 62 percent of patients with IBD were accepted at standard rates. A small number of Crohn's patients had to pay an extra premium. However, about 90 percent of IBD patients applying for group drug plans were successful.

There were several limitations to the study, but it certainly gives you some idea of how insurable people with IBD are. Gastroenterologists are generally aware that many IBD patients must apply to several different companies before they are accepted. When their patients apply for insurance, doctors should point out that these patients are "good citizens" – they have not lost time from work, are able to participate in community activities, and have not had much disability – if that is the case.

Patients who are rejected for one type of insurance often neglect to apply for any other type. Representatives of the insurance industry have pointed out that some of the rejections have nothing to do with the diagnosis of IBD, and are related to other factors. Crohn's and colitis foundations or societies may be very helpful by directing patients to companies that deal with large numbers of patients with IBD.

Unquestionably, disability and premature death due to IBD have decreased significantly in the past 50 years. From the doctors' point of view, the difference in life expectancy between most sufferers of IBD and the general population is minor. Yet this minor difference is important to the insurance companies, who are, after all, in business.

A Strategy for Insurance Applications

Don't be discouraged from applying for insurance just because you have been rejected for one type. And don't give up because you have been rejected by one company; consult your local Crohn's and colitis organization for guidance.

If you have Crohn's disease and you've had a flare-up or surgery, it's probably a good idea to wait at least six months before applying for insurance. The longer you go without active disease, the greater the likelihood of getting regular insurance with no extra premium.

Since it is somewhat difficult for people with Crohn's disease to acquire benefits, it is important to try to stay at the same job. Before you do change employment, consider carefully whether your benefits are transferable.

Looking
Ahead

Research into causes and treatments of IBD continues on many fronts. One exciting area of current research is the use of genetic engineering in laboratory animals. It is possible to create individual immunological defects – known as "gene knockout" models – to allow researchers to study one particular aspect of the immune reaction at a time.

Drug researchers are continuing to search for steroids and other drugs that act locally in the intestine and then promptly become inactivated, so that side effects are reduced. As always, chance observations will be pursued. One recent report was about an ulcerative colitis patient who needed the anticoagulant (blood thinner) heparin for a blood clot in his leg. His colitis improved dramatically when the heparin was started. His doctors treated some other patients, who had a similar response. Further studies are underway.

The role of laparoscopic surgery (using multiple little incisions instead of one big one) in IBD has yet to be determined. Small-bowel transplantation is in its infancy. However, there have now been several successful cases with long-term survival. As this procedure becomes more successful, it will represent an important step forward for patients with small-bowel

Crohn's disease who now require multiple resections, and for those who are already severely disabled because of a surgically shortened small bowel.

Cancer researchers are using molecular genetics and related technology to look for blood or tissue tests that may replace surveillance colonoscopy.

There is every reason to be optimistic that the causes of IBD will be found someday, and we can expect that such discoveries will lead to improved treatments and, ultimately, to cures.

Some Drugs Commonly Used by IBD Patients

Many drugs are used to treat IBD and its complications; the table on the facing page focuses on those that relate most specifically to IBD. Note that some are available as generic ("no-name") products.

Drug Type	Generic Names	Brand Names
Source of 5-ASA	sulfasalazine	Azulfidine*, Azulfidine EN-tabs*, Salazopyrint, Salazopyrin EN-tabs+, S.A.S.+, SAS*
	5-aminosalicylate (5-ASA, mesalamine, mesalazine, olsalazine)	Asacol, Dipentum, Mesasal+, Pentasa, Quintasa+, Rowasa*, Salofalk+
Glucocorticosteroids	prednisone	Deltasone, Liquid Pred Syrup*, Prednicen-N*, Sterapred*, Winpred+
	hydrocortisone	Cortenema, Cortifoam, Cortiment Forte+
	betamethasone	Betnesol+, Celestone Soluspan*
	tixocortol	Rectovalone+
	budesonide	Entocort+
Immunosuppressives	azathioprine	Imuran
	6-mercaptopurine	Purinethol
	methotrexate	Rheumatrex
	cyclosporine, cyclosporine A	Sandimmune, Neoral*
Unclassified topicals	lidocaine	Xylocaine
	cromolyn	Gastrocrom*, Nalcrom+
Antidiarrheals	codeine	——
	diphenoxylate	Lomotil
	loperamide	Imodium, Pepto Diarrhea Control*
Bowel cleanout products	polyethylene glycol-electrolyte solution	Colyte, GoLytely, Lyteprep+, Peglyte
	sodium phosphate solution	Fleet Phosphosoda, PMS-Phosphates Solution
Antibiotics	ciprofloxacin	Cipro
	metronidazole	Flagyl, Protostat*, Trikacide+
Lactose digestive enzymes	lactase	Dairyaid+, Lactaid, Lactrol*, Prolactase+

* Available only in U.S.A.
+ Available only in Canada.

Glossary

Abdominoperineal resection of the rectum: an operation to remove the rectum and anus; it requires incisions in both the abdomen and the perineum.

Abscess: a localized collection of pus (dead cells and a mixture of live and dead bacteria).

Acute: of rapid onset and short duration.

Adenocarcinoma: any cancer originating in glandular tissues such as those found in the gastrointestinal tract.

Adhesions: bands of scar tissue that are usually a result of surgery, and connect the area of surgery to another structure such as a section of intestine, or the peritoneum.

Anal canal: the channel connecting the rectum to the outside world.

Anal sphincter: a ring of muscle surrounding the anal canal, controlling the opening and closing of the anus.

Anastomosis: a surgically created connection of separate or severed tubular hollow organs.

Anemia: abnormally low level of red blood cells or hemoglobin in the blood.

Anus: the lower opening of the anal canal.

Appliance: the plastic bag used to collect stool coming out of an ileostomy or colostomy.

ASA: acetylsalicylic acid, also called aspirin in the U.S.

Ascending colon: section of colon running from the ileocecal valve to the hepatic flexure.

Aylett procedure: an operation used for ulcerative colitis in the 1950s, involving removal of the colon and attachment of the ileum to the rectum.

Barium enema: an X-ray examination of the colon, and sometimes the end of the ileum, using a suspension of barium sulfate, which appears white on X-ray film.

Biliary: pertaining to bile, a fluid that delivers bile salts to the small intestine to help digestion of fat, and carries some toxins and waste from the liver into the bowel; the bile ducts ("biliary tree") extend from inside the liver to the duodenum.

Biopsy: a tissue sample removed for examination under a microscope. An entire area of tissue may be removed, or only a little bit.

Although biopsies are often taken to look for cancer, many other tissue abnormalities are also diagnosed through biopsy.

Brooke ileostomy: most commonly used form of ileostomy, invented by British surgeon Bryan Brooke. *See* **Ileostomy**.

CAT scan: computerized axial tomography, which takes X-rays of "slices" of the body; also known as CT scan.

CD: Crohn's disease.

Cecum: a large, blind pouch, forming the beginning of the colon on the lower right side of the abdomen, where the appendix is.

Chronic: lasting for a long time or frequently recurring.

Colectomy: surgical removal of part or all of the colon; often specified as **total** (including the rectum; also called "proctocolectomy"), or **subtotal** (excluding the rectum).

Colitis: inflammation of the colon.

Colon: the large intestine (or

large bowel), extending from the cecum to the rectum, though the rectum is often referred to separately.

Colonoscopy: an examination of the colon with a flexible instrument inserted into the rectum.

Constipation: bowel movements that are harder or less frequent than normal; may also refer to passage of an inadequate volume of stool.

CT scan: *see* **CAT scan.**

Cyclosporine: an immunosuppressive drug best known for preventing rejection of transplanted organs; lower doses have been studied in patients with IBD.

Descending colon: part of the colon running down the left side, from the splenic flexure to the sigmoid colon.

Diarrhea: bowel movements that are softer, looser, or more frequent than normal.

Duodenum: the first part of the small intestine, starting at the lower end of the stomach and extending to the jejunum.

Elemental diet: a sterilized manufactured diet including protein (as amino acids) and carbohydrate (as glucose) and vitamins, minerals, and a small amount of fat. This diet requires little or no digestion.

Endoscope: an instrument used to examine the inside of a part of the body.

Enteral diet: Strictly speaking, any diet taken by mouth, as opposed to a parenteral diet, which is administered intravenously. But the term is applied to a sterilized manufactured liquid diet which may be drunk or administered through a tube into the stomach or intestine.

Enteritis: inflammation of the small intestine.

Enteroscopy: examination of the small intestine with an endoscope.

Enterostomal therapist: a nurse who specializes in the care of ostomies and some of their complications; also known as an ET.

Enzymes: proteins or conjugated proteins, produced by

living organisms, which speed chemical reactions such as the digestion or breakdown of other substances.

Esophagogastroduodenoscopy: examination of the esophagus, stomach, and duodenum with an endoscope; also known as OGD or EGD.

Esophagus: the swallowing tube, a muscular, tube-like structure that propels food from the throat into the stomach.

False urge: a strong but mistaken feeling that a bowel movement is going to occur; a symptom of rectal inflammation.

Feces: *see* **Stool.**

Fissure: a break in surface tissue, such as skin or mucosa; may be superficial, as in an anal fissure (a tear in the skin of the anal canal), or a deep, crack-like ulcer extending into the wall of the GI tract, as in Crohn's disease.

Fistula: an abnormal connection between two hollow structures (e.g., two segments of intestine, or a segment of intestine and the bladder), or between a hollow structure and the skin surface.

5-ASA: the drug 5-aminosalicylate.

Gastroenterologist: a medical specialist in the diagnosis and treatment of diseases of the stomach, intestines and associated organs (gastrointestinal tract).

Gastrointestinal tract: the mouth, esophagus, stomach, small intestine, large intestine (colon), rectum, anus, liver, biliary system, and pancreas.

GI tract: gastrointestinal tract.

Glucocorticoids: a family of steroid hormones, both synthetic and naturally occurring, that have anti-inflammatory properties.

Growth failure: an effect that any chronic disease may have on a child who has not finished growing. Growth is usually slowed, but may stop completely; reduced activity of the disease, especially in combination with improved nutrition, usually corrects the problem.

Hepatic flexure: a sharp bend in the colon just below the liver, where the ascending colon becomes the transverse colon.

IBD: inflammatory bowel disease, which includes Crohn's disease and ulcerative colitis.

Ileitis: any inflammation of the ileum, although the term is often used as a synonym for Crohn's disease of the ileum.

Ileocecal valve: short area of muscle thickening located where the ileum joins the colon, which controls the release of the fluid contents of the ileum into the colon.

Ileostomy: surgically created opening from the ileum to the abdominal surface, to allow stool to pass from the body into a plastic bag.

Ileum: last portion of the small intestine, extending from the jejunum to the cecum.

Immunosuppressives: a group of medications whose common characteristic is that they reduce activity of

the immune system.

Inflammation: a localized protective reaction to injury or infection, characterized by pain, swelling, redness, heat and sometimes loss of function.

Irritable bowel syndrome (IBS): a disorder of the GI tract usually involving an abnormal bowel habit and abdominal discomfort. IBS can mimic some features of Crohn's disease but does not usually cause weight loss.

Jejunum: upper portion of the small intestine, connecting the duodenum to the ileum.

Kock ileostomy: an ileostomy that allows stool to be collected in an internal reservoir, called a Kock pouch, instead of an external bag; also known as a "continent ileostomy."

Kock pouch: a reservoir for stool, surgically constructed from the ileum; *see* **Kock ileostomy.**

Lactase: an enzyme in the mucosa (inner lining) of the

small intestine that breaks down lactose into two simpler sugars, glucose and galactose.

Lactose: a sugar in dairy products, also found in some processed foods and medications.

Lactose intolerance: a partial or complete inability to digest lactose, generally resulting in abdominal pain, excess lower bowel gas, and sometimes diarrhea; also known as "lactase deficiency."

Lesion: a localized pathological change or injury to body tissue; a cancer is a lesion, and so is a scratch.

Leukocyte scan: a test using radioactively labeled white blood cells (leukocytes) to locate areas of inflammation.

Liquid-diet therapy: a treatment for Crohn's disease using a diet consisting entirely of sterilized liquids, mostly manufactured high-energy products; sometimes used as a nutritional source for people with ulcerative colitis, but it is not a treatment on its own.

Lymphoma: cancer arising in lymphoid tissue, which is present in many locations throughout the body, mainly as lymph glands, and is part of the immune system.

Mesentery: a fan-shaped piece of tissue that acts like a sling, holding the small intestine. Within this sling are lymph glands, fat, and blood vessels.

Modular-diet product: a manufactured product that supplies a single nutrient.

Mucosa: the inner lining of any hollow structure in the body.

Mucous fistula: a surgically created connection between part of the GI tract and the skin; it differs from an ostomy in that the portion of intestine leading to the mucous fistula is disconnected from the flow of bowel contents.

Mucus: nature's lubricant, normally produced by glands of the mucosa.

Osmosis: diffusion of a fluid across a membrane.

Ostomy: surgically created connection between two

portions of the GI tract, or between a portion carrying bowel contents and the skin.

Parenteral: entering the body by a route other than the GI tract, such as by intravenous or intramuscular injection.

Parenteral nutrition: a technique of supplying nutrition directly into the bloodstream, bypassing the intestine.

Pelvic pouch: a reservoir surgically constructed from the ileum, as a substitute for the rectum.

Perforation: a hole right through the wall of a hollow structure.

Peri-anal: around the anus, but the term is also used to refer to the area within the anal canal.

Perineum: the area between the anus and the posterior boundery of the genitals.

Peritoneum: a thin, tough membrane lining the abdominal cavity and folding inward to enclose some of the abdominal organs.

Peritonitis: inflammation of the peritoneum.

Phlegmon: an infected, inflamed mass of tissue.

PN: parenteral nutrition (*see* **Parenteral**).

Polymeric diet: a synthetic diet that contains food components in forms requiring at least some digestion (*see* **Elemental diet**).

Pouchitis: inflammation of either a Kock pouch or a pelvic pouch.

Proctocolectomy: *see* **Colectomy**.

Proctoscopy: examination of the rectum with an endoscope.

Rectum: the last part of the colon, extending from the sigmoid colon to the anal canal.

Resection: surgical removal of an organ or part of an organ.

Serosa: the outer lining of the GI tract, present everywhere except in the esophagus and the lower half of the rectum.

Short-bowel syndrome: a condition of chronic diarrhea and reduced absorption of food, due to surgical removal of a major portion of the small intestine.

Sigmoid colon: part of the colon connecting the descending colon to the rectum.

Sigmoidoscopy: examination of the rectum and sigmoid colon with an endoscope; may include some or all of the descending colon, and some of the transverse colon.

Sign: a finding made during the course of a physical examination, such as an enlarged liver.

Small-bowel enema: an X-ray examination of the small intestine in which a radiologist injects a suspension of barium sulfate through a small plastic tube which has been inserted into the intestine through the nose.

Small-bowel series: an X-ray examination of the small intestine in which the patient drinks a suspension of barium sulfate.

Sphincter: a ring of muscle that opens and closes, to control the passage of something.

Splenic flexure: part of the colon just below the spleen, where the transverse colon turns abruptly to become the descending colon.

Steroids: commonly used to refer to a large number of hormones with a similar chemical structure. They include glucocorticoid steroids (which reduce inflammation), male sex hormones (such as the so-called anabolic steroids sometimes misused by athletes), female sex hormones, and others.

Stoma: the surgically constructed opening of an ostomy.

Stool: a collective term for the various components discharged at the end of the GI tract. Whether this material comes out of the rectum, a colostomy, or an ileostomy, it is still called stool.

Stricture: an abnormal area of narrowing of a hollow organ or structure.

Strictureplasty: a surgical technique that widens an area of narrowing, instead of removing it; also known as "stricturoplasty."

Suppository: rapidly dissolving form of solid medication

that is inserted through the anus into the rectum.
Symptom: something abnormal perceived by the patient, such as fatigue or pain.

Tenesmus: an intense urge to have a bowel movement, relieved partially or not at all by the passage of material from the rectum, whether it is stool, blood, or gas; frequently associated with an inability to pass anything. Tenesmus is a symptom of rectal inflammation.
Topical: medication applied directly to the area affected; a suppository is an example.
Toxic megacolon: the most serious complication of an attack of acute colitis. Some or all of the colon becomes paralyzed, and swells up with gas, stretching the wall.
TPN: total parenteral nutrition; *see* **Parenteral.**
Trace elements: elements required by the body in very tiny amounts, such as zinc and chromium.
Transverse colon: part of the colon running across the upper abdomen, from the hepatic flexure to the splenic flexure.

UC: ulcerative colitis.
Ulcer: a break in a lining; an open sore on an arm is a skin ulcer, for example. The ulcers of the small bowel or colon that occur in ulcerative colitis or Crohn's disease have nothing to do with duodenal or stomach ulcers.
Ulcerative proctitis: ulcerative colitis that only involves the rectum.
Ultrasound: a technique for examining tissues using sound waves.
Upper GI series: X-ray examination of the esophagus, stomach, and duodenum; the patient drinks a suspension of barium sulfate, and several X-rays are taken.

Further Resources

Organizations

There are chapters of the Crohn's and Colitis Foundation and the United Ostomy Association across Canada; check your telephone book for your local chapter.

Canada

Crohn's and Colitis Foundation of Canada
21 St. Clair Avenue E., Suite 301
Toronto, Ontario M4T 1L9
(416) 920-5035
Toll-free 1-800-387-1479
Fax: (416) 929-0364
www.ccfc.ca

United Ostomy Association of Canada Inc.
P.O. Box 825, 50 Charles Street E.
Toronto, Ontario M4Y 2N7
(416) 595-5452
Toll-free 1-888-969-9698
Fax: (416) 595-9924
www3.ns.sympatico.ca/canada.ostomy/

United States
Crohn's and Colitis Foundation of America
386 Park Avenue S., 17th Floor
New York, New York 10016
(212) 685-3440
Fax: (212) 779-4098
www.ccfa.org

United Ostomy Association of America
19772 MacArthur Blvd., Suite 200
Irvine, California 92612
(949) 660-8624
Toll-free 1-800-826-0826
Fax: (949) 660-9262
www.uoa.org

Books

Greenwood, Jan K. *The IBD Nutrition Book*. New York: John Wiley & Sons, 1992.

Jonowitz, Henry D. *Good Food for Bad Stomachs*. New York: Oxford University Press, 1998.

McFarlane, Donna. *Division of Surgery*. Toronto: Women's Press, 1994.

Meyer, Kathleen. *How to Shit in the Woods*. Berkeley, California: Ten Speed Press, 1994.

Scala, Dr. James. *The New Eating Right for a Bad Gut*. New York: Plume, 2000.

Zukerman, Eugenia, and Julie Ingelfinger. *Coping with Prednisone and Other Cortisone-Related Medicines*. New York: St. Martin's Press, 1998.

Index

NOTE: Page numbers in italics refer to illustrations.

abdominal cavity, lining of. *See* peritoneum; peritonitis
abdominal fullness, 30, 39, 53. *See also* bloating
abdominal pain: and bowel obstruction, 115, 140, 141; and colonoscopy, 30; and Crohn's disease, 22, 24, 25, 26, 31, 82, 136; and diet, 38, 39, 46; and drugs, 64, 85; and heartburn, 91, 92; and IBS, 12; and ileostomies, 103, 106; and kidney stones, 154; and liquid diets, 53; as medical emergency, 139, 182; and quality-of-life index, 174; and toxic megacolon, 139; and ulcerative colitis, 20–21
abdominal swelling, 26–27, 31
abdominoperineal resection, 99
abortion, 170, 171
abscesses (boils), 16, 27, 31, 127–32, *129*,141; abdominal, 128, 130; chronic, 131, 132; diagnosing, 34; drainage of, 113, 128, *129*, 130, 142; formation of, 127–28,

141; intestinal, 75; in liver, 75; and perforations, 141; peri-anal, 128, 130, 132, 143; and postoperative leak, 113; recurrence of, 132; surgery for, 114, 124, 127, 130–32; treatment of, 128–32
acetaminophen, 90, 91
acetylsalicylic acid. *See* ASA
adhesions, 132, 134
adolescents. *See* puberty; teens
age: at start of IBD, *v*, 9, 135, 160, 173, 176; and surgery, 107–8, 166
air-contrast barium enema, 30–31
alcohol, 76–77
allergic reactions, 62, 64, 79, 83–84, 91, 93
amino acids, 55
ampicillin, 75
amyloidosis, 154–55
anal canal, 4, 65, 87, 111, 142, 143
anal fissures, 85–87, 143
analgesics, 89–91
anal itching, 87, 89, 143
anal pain/bleeding, 65, 113, 142
anal sphincter, 86, 89, 107, 113, 143
anal strictures, 143–44

anal ulcers, 143
anastomosis, 100, 112, 113, 118, 123, 126; ileo-anal, 107–14; ileorectal, 103, 122, 126
ANCA (antineutrophil cytoplasmic antibodies), 11
anemia, 62, 92, 144–45
anger, 174, 176–77
ankles, 68, 147
ankylosing spondylitis (AS), 11, 147
anorexia nervosa, 136
antibacterials, 61
antibiotics, 22, 74–78, 91–92, 171, 172; colitis associated with, 22, 91–92; and complications of IBD, 132, 142, 149; and Crohn's disease, 61, 72, 74, 75–78; and postoperative complications, 106, 112, 113; and pregnancy, 170; side effects of, 22; and steroids, 68; and ulcerative colitis, 74–75
antibodies, 11, 13–14, 81
anticoagulants, 157
antidiarrheals, 82–83, 111, 124, 153, 170, 171, 178–79
antifungal ointments, 103
anti-inflammatory drugs. *See* drugs, anti-inflammatory; NSAIDs; steroids
anus, 2, 4; fistulas at/near, 75, 132, 133, 143; removal of (*See* procto-colectomy); and strictures, 143–44; and ulcers, 143.
anxiety, 68, 166, 167, 174
appendix, 2, 3, 16, 23, 26, 119
appetite: decreased, 13, 21, 22, 25, 57, 136; increased, 68
appliance, 100, 106, 107, 113, 123, 166
arthralgia, 146. *See also* joints, pain in
arthritis, *vi*, 60, 61, 62, 90, 91, 146–47
arthropathy, enteropathic, 146
ASA (acetylsalicylic acid), 60, 63, 90.

ascending colon, 2, 3
autoimmune diseases, 13–14
avascular necrosis, 148
Aylett procedure, 103–4
azathioprine, 73, 157, 171

back pain/stiffness, 147, 154
backwash ileitis, 8
bacteria, 4, 61, 124; and antibiotics, 74–75; colonic, 39, 45, 120, 139; and inflammation, 13, 51; and intestinal complications of IBD, 127, 140, 141. *See also* germs
balsalazide, 81
barium enemas, 30–33, 161. *See also* small-bowel enema
barium sulfate, 30, 31, 32
betamethasone, 70
bile acids, 152
bile duct, 152
bile-salt binders, 84–85
bile salts, 84, 120, 153
biliary tree, 151–52
biopsies, 29, 33, 79, 148, 161
birth control, 15, 168
birth defects, 170
bisacodyl, 88
black stools, 93
bladder, 130, 133
bleeding, 19; anal, 65; chronic, 144, 145; sudden/massive, 145, 146, 182; unusual, 63. *See also* blood
blisters, 150
bloating, 39, 82, 83, 85, 115, 141, 174. *See also* abdominal fullness
blockages. *See* obstructions; throm-bosed hemorrhoids
blood: infected (septicemia), 55, 75; in stools, 19, 24, 106, 144, 145. *See also* anemia; bleeding
blood cells, 62–63, 156; counts/scans of, 35, 73, 156,; leukocytes, 35; lymphocytes, 13; red, 62, 144, 145; white, 35, 65, 78, 79, 127, 128

blood clots/clotting, 55, 142, 156–57

blood pressure, 69, 74

blood vessels: abnormal, 14; bleeding, 145, 146; clotting in, 55, 142, 156–57

boils. *See* abscesses

bone biopsies, 148

bone densitometry, 69, 148

bone disease, 43, 69, 147–49

bone marrow, 62–63, 144, 145

bone meal, 44

bones, 43, 69, 148–49

bowel movements: after surgery, 104, 111, 122; frequency of, 86, 174; and iron supplements, 93; irregular, 12; normal, 86; pain during/after, 143; urgency of, 82, 104, 111; wiping after, 87, 89. *See also* constipation; diarrhea; incontinence

bowel obstructions, 115–18, 132, 134, 140, 141–42; diagnosing, 35, 141; and diet, 47, 49, 115, 182; managing, 82, 115, 116, 182; and surgery, 114, 116–18, 124, 132, 134; symptoms of, 115, 140, 141, 182

bowel, twisted, 132, 133

bran, 46, 84

brand-name drugs, 64

breastfeeding, 171–72

broad-spectrum antibiotics, 74–75

Brooke (end) ileostomy, 101–3, *102*, 104, 107–13 *passim*, 122, 140, 166

bruising, 63, 68

budesonide, 70, 71

bulk formers, 83–84

B$_{12}$vitamins, 62, 85, 121, 144, 145

bypass, exclusion, 161

caesarian sections, 168

caffeine, 22, 78

calcium, 42–44, 94, 148

calcium oxalate, 153, 154

calories, 42

cancer, *vi*, 157, 159–63, 188; colon, 100, 113–14, 159, 160; Crohn's disease and, 157, 159, 160–61, 163, 173; of gallbladder or bile duct, 152; and immunosuppressives, 71, 73; proctitis and, 160, 162; risk of, 73, 113, 160–61, 173; screening for, 30, 122, 161–63; small-bowel, 157, 159, 160–61, 163; and surgery, 161; symptoms/signs of, 161; ulcerative colitis and, 113, 157, 159, 160, 162, 163

cankers (mouth sores), 74, 149–50

casein, 49

cataracts, 69

CAT (CT) scans, 34–35, 130

cavities, dental, 149–50

cecum, 2, 3

cefazolin, 75

cell changes (dysplasia), 100, 161, 162

cephalexin, 76

cereal fiber, 46

chest pain, 25. *See also* heartburn

children/young people and IBD, 52, 69, 135–38, 160, 171–72, 176–77, 180–81

chills, 21, 73

cholesterol, 153

cholestyramine, 85, 120

chromium, 94

chronic continuous colitis, 21, 67

cimetidine, 92

ciprofloxacin, 75, 76, 77–78, 171, 172

cirrhosis of the liver, 47, 74

clear fluid diets, 47–48, 54, 88, 115, 182

closed ileostomy, 108

clots/clotting, 55, 142, 156–57

codeine, 82, 83, 85, 171

colchicine, 155

colectomy, 99, 126, 172; near-total, 99–100, 110, 167; subtotal (*See* subtotal colectomy); total (*See* proctocolectomy)

colitis, 55, 64, 66, 79, 88–89, 113, 162, 172; antibiotic-associated, 22, 91–92; chronic continuous, 21, 67; idiopathic ulcerative, 6; indeterminate, 6, 114; infectious, 12; NSAID, 90; total, 162; toxic, 141. *See also* Crohn's disease of the colon (Crohn's colitis); proctitis; ulcerative colitis

colon, *v*, 2; 90, 124, 162, *190–91*; ascending, 2, 3; bacteria in, 39, 45, 120, 139; and bile salts, 84; cancer of, 100, 113–14, 159, 160; descending, 2, 4; examining, 30–31; lining of (*See* mucosa); obstruction in (*See* bowel obstructions); perforation of, 91, 140; polyps in, 160; sigmoid (*See* sigmoid colon); surgery involving (*See* colectomy; colostomy; resection); transverse, 2, 4. *See also* colitis; colostomy; Crohn's disease of the colon; toxic megacolon; ulcerative colitis

colonic-lavage solutions, 88

colonoscopy, 30, 31, 32–33, 122, 161–63

colostomy, *100*, 118, 123

complications: of IBD (intestinal), 135, 139–46; of IBD (nonintestinal), 135, 146–58; postoperative, 106, 110, 111–14, 132, 134, 145, 153, 166, 173

confined perforations, 127, 141

congenital abnormalities, 170

conjunctivitis, 155

constipation, 19, 22, 86, 88–89, 142, 182; in children, 136; as side effect, 44, 76, 82, 85, 93

contact lenses, 63

continent ileostomy. *See* Kock ileostomy

contraception, 15, 168

coping strategies, 177–79

cortisol, 66, 69–70

cortisone, 60, 66

cramps. *See* abdominal pain

Crohn's colitis. *See* Crohn's disease of the colon

Crohn's disease of the colon (Crohn's colitis), 33, 51, 140; and cancer, 157, 159, 160, 162, 163; drugs and, 75–76, 77; recurrence of, 125, 126–27; surgery for, 122–23, 124–25, 126–27; symptoms of, 24

Crohn's disease of the ileum, 31–33, 77, 84–85, 118–21, 126, 127, 145, 153–54

Crohn's disease of the ileum and colon, 8, 25, 31, 123, 125, 126, 127

cromolyn enemas, 79

cures, *v*, 95–96

cyclosporine, 74, 152

cystic fibrosis, 11

death, 169, 172–73

dehydration, 103, 156

delayed growth/puberty, 68, 136, 137

denial, 180

dental cavities, 149–50

dependency, 176

depression, 68, 138, 174

descending colon, 2, 4

dextran, 94

diabetes mellitus, 69

dialysis, 155

diarrhea: bile-salt, 120; and bowel obstruction, 140; and cortisol, 70; and Crohn's disease, 22, 24, 31, 82, 136; and diet, 38, 39, 40, 44–45, 46, 52, 69, 87, 94; drugs for (*See* antidiarrheals; bile-salt binders; bulk formers; sulfasalazine); effects of, 87, 103, 142, 156; non-IBD causes of, 22; and quality of life, 165, 167, 174, 175; as side effect of drugs, 22,

64, 66, 76, 78, 91, 93, 171; as
    side effect of surgery, 118, 120,
    124, 167; and toxic megacolon,
    139; and ulcerative colitis, 19
diclofenac, 90
dietary fiber (roughage), 4–5, 15, 22,
    44–46, 56, 86, 87, 103, 107, 182
dietitians, 37, 43, 58
diet(s), 37–58, 170; clear fluid,
    47–48, 54, 88, 115, 182; and
    Crohn's disease, 37, 45–46, 47,
    49, 51, 56; elemental, 49–54;
    enteral, 94, 116, 137, 170; full
    fluid, 48–49; high-iron, 93, 95;
    liquid, 49–54, 137; low-oxalate,
    153–54; older people and, 48,
    57–58; polymeric, 49–54; as pos-
    sible cause of IBD, 16–17; and
    reduction of IBD symptoms, 38,
    39, 47, 49, 87, 115, 182; side
    effects of, 39, 44–45, 46, 49, 50,
    52, 53, 56, 57, 58, 69, 93, 103,
    107, 167; and ulcerative colitis,
    50; unnecessary restrictions in,
    37, 56–58, 138. *See also* fat in
    diet; dietary fiber; lactose intoler-
    ance; malnutrition; nutrition; PN;
    TPN
dilatation, 112, 116, 144. *See also*
    stretching
diphenoxylate, 82, 83, 85, 111, 153,
    171
discouragement, 174
dizziness, 81, 82
drainage: of abscess (boil), 113, 128,
    129, 130, 142; of fistulous tract,
    131, 132
dreams, 78, 81
drowsiness, 82
drug plans, 78, 79, 81, 83, 179, 185.
    See also insurance
duodenal ulcers, 25, 69, 90, 91
duodenum, 1, 2, 3; Crohn's disease
    of the, 25, 33, 123, 133
dysplasia, 100, 161, 162

EGD, 33
ejaculation, retrograde, 112, 167
electrolyte solutions, 30
elemental diets, 49–54
emergencies, medical, 139, 140, 141,
    182, 183
emergency surgery, 140, 141, 146
emotions, 12, 69, 70, 136, 174
employment. *See* work/school
end ileostomy. *See* Brooke ileostomy
endoscope, 116, 161, 162
endoscopic recurrence, 125
endoscopic retrograde cholangio-
    pancreatography (ERCP), 152
enemas, 74, 125; barium, 30–33,
    161; and constipation, 88; cro-
    molyn, 79; 5-ASA, 65, 66, 171,
    182; lidocaine, 78–79; risks/side
    effects of, 59, 78–79, 88; short-
    chain fatty acid, 79; small-bowel,
    32; steroid, 67, 70, 71, 182;
    sulfasalazine, 63; tapwater, 88
enteral diets, 94, 116, 137, 170
enteritis, 6, 22
enteropathic arthropathy, 146
enteroscopy, 33, 163
enterostomal therapists, 103
enzymes, 38
eosinophils, 79
epileptic seizures, 79
episcleritis, 155–56
erythema nodosum, 150
erythromycin, 76
esophagitis, reflux, 92
esophagogastroduodenoscopy
    (OGD; EGD), 33
esophagus, 1, *2*, *124*; Crohn's
    disease of the, 25, 33, 124
ethnicity/race, 9–10, 39–40
euphoria, 68
exclusion bypass, 161
exercise, 43, 148, 157, 178
eye problems, 69, 155–56

fallopian tubes, 167
false urge, 19–20, 24

family history. *See* genetic predisposition
famotidine, 92
fat in diet, 46–47, 48, 49, 50, 57, 84–85, 120, 153
fatigue, 22, 70, 174; taste, 53, 54
fatty acids: omega-3, 81; short-chain, 15–16, 79
fatty liver, 150
feces, 4. *See also* stool(s)
feet, 76
ferrous gluconate, 92
ferrous sulfate, 92, 93
fertility, 63, 167–68. *See also* pregnancy
fetal death/deformity, 169, 170
fever: and allergic reactions to drugs, 62, 64; and blood clots, 156; as medical emergency, 139, 182; as symptom of IBD, 21, 136; as symptom of infection, 73, 113; as symptom of toxic megacolon, 139
fiber. *See* bulk formers; dietary fiber
fish oil, 81
fissures, 85–87, 143
fistulas, 27, 31, 114, 127, 130, *133*, 141–42, and antibiotics, 75; between bowel segments, 130; and diet, 49; formation of, 127, 142; ileo-vesical (ileum-to-bladder), 133; peri-anal, 75, 132, 133, 143; recto-vaginal, 133; recurrence of, 132; to bladder, 130, 133; to skin surface, 130; and surgery, 114, 118, 124, 127, 132, 142; types of, 130, 133; to vagina, 130, 133. *See also* fistulous tracts; mucous fistula of the rectum
fistulous tracts, *131*, 132, *133*. *See also* fistulas
5-ASA (5-aminosalicylate), 22, 60–66, 72, 113, 171, 182, 183; side effects of, 22, 64–65, 157, 171

FK-506, 81
flare-up. *See* recurrence
flexible sigmoidoscopy. *See* sigmoidoscopy
flexure. *See* hepatic flexure; splenic flexure
fluid diets: clear, 47–48, 54, 88, 115, 182; full, 48–49. *See also* liquid diets
fluid intake, 103, 153
fluid loss, 153
fluticasone, 71
folic acid (folate), 46, 62, 85, 144
forcing/straining, 86, 143
4-ASA (4-aminosalicyclate), 81
"free" perforations, 141
free radicals, 16
fructose, 44–45
fruits, 44–46
full fluid diets, 48–49
functional impairment, 174
fungal infections, 102–3

galactose, 38, 39
gallbladder, 2
gallbladder cancer, 152
gallstones, *vi*, 153, 173
gas, 20, 34–35, 174; and bowel obstruction, 140; and diet, 38, 39, 44, 45; as side effect of drugs/surgery, 83, 111; and toxic megacolon, 139–40
gastroenterologists, 31, 32, 114
gastrointestinal (GI) tract, 1–5, *2*, 13–14
gastrojejunostomy, 123, 124
generic drugs, 64, 90
"generic" side effects, 59
genetic engineering, 187
genetic predisposition, 10–12, 160
gentamicin, 75
germs, 92, 127, 128. *See also* bacteria
GI motor meal. *See* small-bowel series
glands, 66, 96, 114
glaucoma, 69

glucocorticoids/glucocorticosteroids *(See* steroids)
glucose, 38, 39, 49
glutamine, 55–56
glycerine suppositories, 88
gold, 22
gout, 155
gouty arthritis, 147
government health plans, 53, 179
granulomatous ileitis/enteritis/colitis, 6
growth failure/delay, 68, 136, 137
gum infections, 149–50
gum, nicotine, 80–81

H-2 blockers, 92
hair, 65, 68
hands, shaking of, 81
headaches, 63, 64, 76–77, 90, 156
health plans, 53, 179. *See also* insurance
heartbeat, rapid/pounding, 77
heartburn, 91, 92
hemolysis, 62
hemorrhage, 144, 145, 146, 182. *See also* bleeding
hemorrhoids, 27, 85–87, 142, 143
heparin, 187
hepatic flexure, 2, 3
hepatitis, 62
high blood pressure, 69, 74
high-glutamine products, 55–56
histamine-2-receptor antagonists, 92
hives, 62, 64, 82
hospitalization, 176, 178, 179
HPN (home parenteral nutrition), 55
hydrocortisone, 70, 86, 113, 182
hydronephrosis, 154
hyperbaric oxygen, 81

IBD. *See* inflammatory bowel disease
IBS. *See* irritable bowel syndrome
ibuprofen, 90
idiopathic ulcerative colitis, 6
ileal disease. *See* Crohn's disease of the ileum; ileitis; ileum

ileal pouch. *See* Kock pouch
ileitis, 6, 8, 77, 154. *See also* Crohn's disease of the ileum
ileo-anal anastomosis, 107–14, *108*
ileocecal valve, 2, 3, 118, 120
ileorectal anastomosis, 103, 122, 126
ileostomy, 100–114, 126. *See also* Brooke (end) ileostomy; Kock (continent) ileostomy
ileo-vesical (ileum-to-bladder) fistulas, *133*
ileum, 2, 3; examining, 30, 31–32; and nutrient absorption, 56, 84, 121, 148, 153; surgery involving (*See* ileostomy; resection). *See also* Crohn's disease of the ileum; Crohn's disease of the ileum and colon; ileitis; ileocecal valve
immobility, 156–57
immunity/immune response, 13–14, 69, 127
immunoglobulin infusions, 81
immunosuppressives, 71–74, 152, 170, 171, 172
impotence, 112, 166, 167
incontinence, 104, 107, 110, 111–12, 165, 167
indeterminate colitis, 6, 114
indigestion, 76, 91
indium-111, 35
infants, 135, 171–72. *See also* children
infections: and abscesses (boils), 127–28; of blood (septicemia), 55, 75; and diagnosing IBD, 22, 29; fungal, 102–3; gum, 149–50; and ileostomies, 102, 113; and immunosuppressives, 73; in liver, 152; as possible cause of IBD, 12, 17; and steroids, 69; symptoms of, 73, 113
infectious colitis, 12
infertility, 63, 167–68
inflammation, 5, 62, 144, 155–56, 170; at anastomosis, 113; of bile

duct, 152; of bowel (*See* inflammatory bowel disease); of joints (*See* arthritis); of liver, 62; of pancreas, 64; of peritoneum (*See* peritonitis); of pouch (*See* pouchitis); of tendons, 78

inflammatory bowel disease (IBD): causes of, 10–17; complications of (*See under* complications); diagnosing, 19, 29–35, 135–36; frequency of, 9–10; managing/living with, *vi*, 165–86; overview of, 5–8.

inner lining of colon. *See* mucosa

insomnia, 68, 78

insurance, 53, 179, 184–86. *See also* drug plans; health plans

intercourse. *See* sexual activity

interleukins, 81

intestinal complications of IBD, 135, 139–46

intestinal tuberculosis, 12, 22

intestine: large (*See* colon); small (*See* small bowel)

ipsalazide, 81

iron, 46, 92–94, 95, 144–45

irritable bowel syndrome (IBS), 12, 22, 23–24, 168

ischemic disease of the intestine, 22

itching: anal, 87, 89, 143; with rash (hives), 62, 64, 82

IV (intravenous) feeding, 178. *See also* PN

jaundice, 170

jejunum, 2, 3, 56, 121, 124; Crohn's disease of the, 33, 121

joints: hip, 148; inflamed (*See* arthritis); knee, 148; large, 147; pain in, 90–91, 146–47 (*See also* arthritis); sacroiliac, 147; of spine, 147; stiffness in, 69

ketoprofen, 90

kidney damage/failure, 65, 74, 90, 154, 155

kidney stones, *vi*, 44, 103, 153–54, 173

kilocalories, 42

knees, 147, 148

Kock (continent) ileostomy, 100, 104–7, *105*, 112, 113, 166

Kock pouch, 104–7, *105*, 112, 113

lactase, 38–39, 41, 42

lactose intolerance, 22, *38*, 38–44, 50, 59, 69, 136

lansoprazole, 92

laparoscopic surgery, 187

large bowel/intestine. *See* colon

laxatives/laxative effects, 44–45, 46, 88–89, 120

leakage. *See* postoperative leakage

legs, 76, 150, 156

leukocyte scan, 35

lidocaine, 78–79, 149

life expectancy, 152, 172–73, 186

light-headedness, 70, 81

lining: of abdominal cavity (*See* peritoneum); of bowel (*See* mucosa); of eye, 155

liquid diets, 49–54, 137. *See also* fluid diets

liver, 2, 120; damage/disease in, 47, 74, 75, 90, 150–52; inflamed (hepatitis), 62. *See also* bile salts

long-chain triglycerides, 49

loop ileostomy, 108, 110

loperamide, 82–83, 85, 111, 153, 171

low-oxalate diets, 153–54

lymphocytes, 13

magnesium citrate, 30

maintenance therapy, 65, 67, 183

malignancy. *See* cancer

malnutrition, 15–16, 68, 69, 107, 144, 150, 158, 167. *See also* nutritional deficiencies

marrow aplasia, 62–63

MCT (medium-chain triglyceride), 47, 49, 50

measles, 14

medical emergencies, 139, 140, 141, 182, 183
megacolon, toxic, 55, 139–40, 141
menstruation, 168
mesalamine, 65
mesalazine, 65
mesentery, 8
metallic taste, 76, 85
methotrexate, 73–74, 152, 171
methyldopa, 22
methylprednisolone, 70
metronidazole, 75–77, 106, 170, 171, 172
milk. *See* lactose intolerance
mineral oil, 88–89, 182
minerals, 46, 49, 94, 96, 158
miscarriages, 168
misoprostol, 91
modular products, 49–54
monoclonal antibodies, 81
mood changes, 68
mouth sores/ulcers, 74, 149–50
mucosa, 8, 13, 15–16, 29, 100, 107, 114, 127, 130
mucous fistula of the rectum, 101, *102*, 108, 109, 140
mucus, 5, 107, 124
multiple sclerosis, 11
muscles: exercising, 157, 178; stiff, 69; weak (*See* weakness)

N-acetyl glucosamine, 96
naproxen, 90
narcotic antidiarrheals, 82, 83, 170
narrowing: of anastomosis, 112; of stomach, 123–24. *See also* bowel obstructions; obstructions; scarring; strictures
nausea: and bowel obstruction, 115, 140, 141; and colonoscopy, 30; and cortisol, 70; and Crohn's disease, 25; as side effect of drugs, 61–62, 64, 74, 76, 77, 78, 81, 82, 85, 91, 93; as side effect of liquid diets, 52, 53; and toxic megacolon, 139

near-total colectomy, 99–100, 110, 167
necrosis, avascular, 148
nerve cells, 78
nerve damage, 76
nervousness. *See* anxiety
nicotine, 80–81
night sweats, 68
nitric oxide, 16
nizatidine, 92
nondrug therapies. *See* diet(s); surgery
nonintestinal complications of IBD, 135, 146–58
nonspecific ulcerative colitis, 6
NSAID colitis, 90
NSAIDs (nonsteroidal anti-inflammatory drugs), 22, 90–91
numbness, 76
nutrition, 48, 57–58, 137, 158; parenteral (*See* PN). *See also* diet(s)
nutritional deficiencies, 15–16, 43, 85, 92, 94, 144–45, 158. *See also* malnutrition

obstructions: bowel (*See* bowel obstructions); of fallopian tubes, 167; and ileostomies, 101; of stomach, 123–24; of ureter, 154
OGD, 33
older people and IBD, 48, 57–58, 107–8
olsalazine, 65
omega-3-fatty-acids, 81
omeprazole, 91, 92
operations, multiple- vs. single-stage, 109–10. *See also* surgery
opium, tincture of, 82, 83
oral contraceptives, 15, 168
organ transplants. *See* transplants
"orthomolecular" medicine, 96
osteonecrosis, 147–48
osteoporosis, 43, 69, 148–49
ostomy, 100, 124–25. *See also* appliance; colostomy; gastrojejunostomy; ileostomy

overprotectiveness, 180–81
oversewn rectum, 122
oxidants, 16
oxygen, hyperbaric, 81
oxygen metabolites, reactive, 16
oxygen radicals, 61, 64
oyster shells, 44

pain: and abscesses (boils), 128, 130;
    anal, 65, 113, 142, 143; back,
    147, 154; chest, 25; eye, 156; and
    intercourse, 166, 167; and iron
    injections, 93; joint, 90–91,
    146–47; pelvic, 113, 125. *See
    also* abdominal pain
painkillers, 89–91
pancreatitis, 64, 73, 157
paregoric, 82, 83
parenteral nutrition. *See* HPN;
    PN; TPN
passive smoking, 15, 135
pelvic pain, 113, 125
pelvic pouch, 107–14, *108*, 167
penicillin, 45
perforations, 91, 140, 141; confined,
    127, 141; "free," 141
peri-anal disease, 27, 77, 123,
    127–32, 142–44. *See also*
    abscesses (boils); fistulas
perineal incision, 122, 123
perineum, 99
peri-operative care, 100
peritoneum, 1, 132
peritonitis, 140
petroleum jelly, 89
phosphate solutions, 30, 88
physical activity/inactivity, 69, 178
physical stress, 69, 70
piles. *See* hemorrhoids
the pill, 15, 168
piroxicam, 90
placebo effect, 94–96, 97
PN (parenteral nutrition), 54, 55.
    See also HPN; TPN
polyethylene glycol (PEG), 88
polymeric diets, 49–54

polyps, 160
postoperative complications. *See
    under* complications
postoperative leakage, 103, 106,
    107, 112–13, 166
potassium, 46, 69
pouch. *See* Kock pouch; pelvic
    pouch
pouchitis, 106, 107, 112
precancerous changes in bowel, 100,
    161, 162
prednisone, 43, 51, 66, 70, 72, 115
prednisone metasulfabenzoate, 71, 81
pregnancy, 107, 168–71. *See also*
    fertility
premature births, 168, 170
proctectomy, 123
proctitis, 64, 78, 160, 162. *See also*
    ulcerative proctitis
proctocolectomy (total colectomy),
    99, 100, 104, 107, 113, 122,
    166–67
protein, 41, 48, 49, 50, 155
PSC (primary sclerosing cholangitis),
    150–52
psoriasis, 11
psyllium seed, 84
puberty, delayed, 68, 136
pus, 113, 127, 128, 129, 141, 143
pyoderma gangrenosum (PG), 150

quality of life, 173–79, 180, 181

race/ethnicity, 9–10, 39–40
radiation enteritis, 22
radicals, free/oxygen, 16, 61, 64
ranitidine, 92
rashes, itchy (hives), 62, 64, 82
reactive oxygen metabolites, 16
rectal foam, 65, 70, 71, 182
recto-vaginal fistulas, *133*
rectum, 2, 4, 5, 29, 124–25;
    colitis/inflammation of, 7, 20 (*See
    also* proctitis); and drugs (*See*
    enemas; rectal foam; supposito-
    ries); examination of, 29; over-

sewn, 122; puncturing, 59, 79;
and surgery, 122, 123, 124–25
(*See also* mucous fistula of the
rectum; proctocolectomy
recurrence, 125, 174
red blood cells, 62, 144, 145
redness, 67, 150, 156
reflux esophagitis, 92
regional enteritis/ileitis, 6
relationships, family/social, 174,
176, 179–81. *See also* sexual
activity
remissions, 95, 169
research, 16–17, 187–88
resection, 100, 116, 118–21, 123,
132; abdominoperineal, 99; and
recurrence of Crohn's disease,
125, 126, 127; side effects of,
118–21, 153–54, 173. *See also*
shortening
residue, 49
rest, 138
retrograde ejaculation, 112, 167
rheumatoid arthritis, 60, 147
risks: of cancer, 113, 160–61, 173;
of dying from IBD, 172–73; of
therapeutic abortion, 170; and
unorthodox therapies, 96–97
"roughage." *See* dietary fiber
rounding, facial, 67

sacroiliac joints, 147
sacroiliitis. *See* ankylosing
spondylitis
salt, 88, 103, 120
scarring, 5, 25, 101, 112, 116, 131,
151–52. *See also* adhesions;
narrowing
Schilling test, 121, 145
school. *See* work/school
sclerosing cholangitis, 150–52, *151*
screening for cancer, 30, 122,
161–63
second-hand smoke, 15, 135
sedation, 30, 32, 33
seizures, 79

self-confidence, 179, 181
self-consciousness, 137–38, 176
self-reliance, 179, 181
septicemia, 55, 75
serosa, 8, 101, *195*
sexual activity/satisfaction, 112,
165–67, 173, 179
shaking of hands, 81
short-bowel syndrome, 49, 55
short-chain fatty acids, 15–16, 79
shortening of bowel, 162. *See also*
resection; short-bowel syndrome
shortness of breath, 77
side effects, 59; of colonoscopy
preparations, 30; of drugs (*See
under specific drug type [e.g.,
antibiotics] or name [e.g.,
metronidazole]*); "generic," 59;
of liquid diets, 52, 53; of surgery,
111–14, 118–21, 123, 124–25,
132, 134
sigmoid colon, 2, 4, 30, 162, 172
sigmoidoscopy, 29, 31, 33, 162, 163
signs: of cancer, 161; of Crohn's
disease, 26–27, 126; of ulcerative
colitis, 21
single-contrast barium enema, 31
sitz baths, 86–87, 89, 128, 132
6-mercaptopurine (6-MP), 72, 73,
157, 171
skin: irritated, 81, 102, 103, 143;
sores/ulcers on, 150; thinning,
68, 87; yellowing, 63
skin conditions/diseases, *vi*, 150
skin tags, 27, 142–43
sleep disturbance, 68, 78, 81, 174
small bowel, 1–3; cancer of, 157,
159, 160–61, 163; perforations
of, 91
small-bowel Crohn's disease, 56, 64,
66, 76, 182; and cancer, 157,
159, 160–61, 163; complications
of, 140, 146; and diet(s), 45–46,
47, 49, 51; and surgery, 116,
125, 126, 173; symptoms of,
22, 23

small-bowel enema, 32
small-bowel series (small-bowel follow-through), 32
small-bowel transplants, 187–88
smoking, 14, 15, 80–81, 126, 135
sodium phosphate solutions, 30, 88
softening: of bones, 69, 148–49; of stools, 85–86, 88
sorbitol, 44–45
sores: mouth, 74, 149–50; skin, 150. *See also* ulcers
sore throat, 73
spasm, anal, 86
spleen, 2, 62
splenic flexure, 2, 4
sterilized liquids. *See* enteral diets
steroids (glucocorticoids/glucocorticosteroids), 66–71, 86, 87, 89, 170, 171, 182; vs. anabolic steroids, 51, 66; and bowel obstructions, 115, 116, 182; and children, 136, 137; vs. immunosuppressives, 72; reducing/stopping, 50–51, 69–70, 109; side effects of, 43, 67–69, 71, 87, 148, 171; and surgery, 109; and toxic megacolon, 140
stiffness, 69, 147
stillbirths, 170
stimulants, 78
stoma, 100
stomach, 1, 2, 124; Crohn's disease of, 25, 33, 123–24; obstructions of, 123–24; ulcers of, 69, 90, 91
stones. *See* gallstones; kidney stones
stool(s): black, 93; blood in, 19, 24, 106, 144, 145; and bowel obstructions, 140; consistency of, 86, 174 (*See also* diarrhea; stool softening); dark, 93; fluid loss in, 153; normal, 4–5; samples of, 29; and skin irritation, 87
stool softening, 85–86, 88
straining/forcing, 86, 143
stress, *v*, 12, 69, 70, 136
stretching: and abscesses (boils),

128, 129; and anal fissures, 143; and hemorrhoids, 143; and strictures, 112, 116, 144
strictureplasty, 116–18, *117*, 121, 123
strictures, 31, 45–46, 112, 140–41, 143–44. *See also* narrowing
subtotal colectomy, *99*, 100–101, 103, 109, 122, 126, 140
sugar, 48, 150. *See also* fructose
sulfa drugs, 61
sulfasalazine, 60–63, 66, 72, 75–76, 144, 157, 167–68, 170, 171
sulindac, 90
sunlight, 43, 148–49
supplements, 85, 93, 94, 145, 148
suppositories: bisacodyl, 88; 5-ASA, 65, 66, 113, 171, 182; glycerine, 88; steroid, 70, 71, 86, 87, 113; sulfasalazine, 63
surgery, 99–134, 173, 174; for abscesses (boils), 114, 124, 127, 130–32; age and, 107–8, 166; and bowel obstructions, 114, 116–18; and cancer risk, 161; for children with IBD, 137; complications of (*See* complications, postoperative); for Crohn's disease, 61, 67, 76, 106, 114–34, 169, 173; emergency, 140, 141, 146; and fertility, 167; and fistulas, 114, 118, 124, 127, 132, 142; laparoscopic, 187; multiple- vs. single-stage, 109–10; and nonintestinal complications of IBD, 148; for peri-anal disease, 127–32; and peritonitis, 140; and pregnancy, 169–70; risk of requiring, 172, 173; and sexual activity, 166; side effects of, 111–14, 118–21, 123, 124–25, 132, 134; and toxic megacolon, 140; for ulcerative colitis, 100–114, 172. *See also under specific operation (e.g., resection)*

surveillance colonoscopy, 30, 122, 161–63

sweats/sweating, 21, 68, 81

swelling: abdominal, 26–27, 31; of ankles, 68; of hands/face, 62, 64; of joints, 147. *See also* abscesses (boils); bowel obstructions

symptoms: of bowel obstruction, 115, 140, 141, 182; of cancer, 161; in children, 135, 136; of Crohn's disease, 21–26, 125–26, 135, 136, 168, 182–83; and drugs, 59–60, 70, 82–94; of IBS, 12, 168; systemic, 174; while traveling, 182–83; of ulcerative colitis, 19–21, 29, 182

tags, skin, 27, 142–43

tapwater enemas, 88

taste, metallic, 76

taste fatigue, 53, 54

teens/young people, 137–38, 176–77, 180

temporary colostomy, 118

tendons, 78

tenesmus, 20

tension. *See* stress

terminal ileitis, 6

tetracycline, 76, 149

therapeutic abortion, 170, 171

thickening: of bowel wall, 34, 115, *115*, 140; of skin tags, 143

three-stage operation, *108*, 109–10

throat ulcers, 149

thrombosed hemorrhoids, 142

tincture of opium, 82, 83

tingling, 76

tixocortol, 70, 71

TLA (T-lymphocyte apheresis), 81

TNF (tumor necrosis factor), 81

tobramycin, 75

tomography, 34

tongue, furry, 76

total colitis, 162

toxic colitis, 141

toxic megacolon, 55, 139–40, 141

TPN (total parenteral nutrition), 54–55, 94, 170

trace elements, 49

transplants, 71, 73, 152, 155, 187–88

transverse colon, 2, 4

traveling, 181–83

triglycerides, 47, 49, 50

tube feeding, 52, 137, 178

tuberculosis, intestinal, 12, 22

twisted bowel, 132, 133

two-stage operation, 110

ulcerative proctitis, 7, 19, 64, 78, 79, 160, 172

ulcers: anal, 143; duodenal, 25, 69, 90, 91; mouth/throat, 74, 149; NSAIDs and, 91; skin, 150; stomach, 69, 90, 91

ultrasound, 34, 130, 154

United Ostomy Association of Canada, 200

unorthodox therapies, 96–97

upper GI series, 33

ureter, obstructed, 154

urge: false, 19–20, 24; importance of not resisting, 125

urgency, 82, 104, 111

uric acid, 153

urinary tract, 154

urine/urinating, 63, 65, 103, 121

ursodeoxycholic acid (UDCA), 152

uveitis, 156

vagina, 130, 133, 166

vegetables, 44–46

viscous lidocaine, 149

vision. *See* eye problems

vitamins, 49, 85, 94, 96, 158; fat-soluble, 89; vitamin A, 46, 85, 89; vitamin B_{12}, 121, 144, 145; vitamin C, 46; vitamin D, 41, 43–44, 85, 89, 148–49; vitamin E, 85, 89; vitamin K, 85, 89. *See also* B vitamins

vomiting, 25, 30, 156; as medical

emergency, 139, 140, 182; as side
effect of drugs, 61, 76, 77, 82, 85

weakness, 68, 70, 174, 178
weight gain, 68, 116, 170, 178
weight loss, 21, 22, 23, 25, 31, 34,
    37, 46, 56, 57, 58, 136, 158
white blood cells, 35, 65, 78, 79,
    127, 128
wiping after bowel movements,
    87, 89
work/school, IBD and, 174, 179–80,
    183–84, 186

X-rays, 31–32, 33, 147, 148, 163.
    See also barium enemas; CAT
    (CT) scans

yellowing of skin, 63
young people, 137–38, 176–77, 180.
    See also children

zinc, 94
zinc oxide, 89

To the Reader

Your Personal Health Series is developed with the Canadian Medical Association and will encompass more than 20 subjects. The first 13 publications are *Migraine, Eyes, Arthritis, Sleep, Crohn's Disease & Ulcerative Colitis, The Complete Breast Book, The Pain Relief Handbook, The Complete Allergy Book, Multiple Sclerosis, Alzheimer's Disease, When a Child Has Diabetes, Epilepsy and Seizures* and *Eating Disorders*. We expect to publish at least three new titles each year.

If you wish to be kept informed about the series, please complete and send us this page (or a photocopy). We will be pleased to send you periodic publication notices on new and forthcoming titles.

Key Porter Books Limited
70 The Esplanade
Toronto, Ontario M5E 1R2 Canada
Telephone (416) 862-7777 • Fax (416) 862-2304

☐ Please keep me informed about *Your Personal Health Series.*

☐ Please ship and bill _____ copy/ies of each new book upon publication.

_____
NAME

_____
AFFILIATION (COMPANY/ASSOCIATION/INSTITUTION/MEDICAL AFFILIATION)

_____
ADDRESS

_____
CITY/TOWN   PROVINCE   POSTAL CODE

PAYMENT BY: ☐ VISA   ☐ MASTERCARD

_____
CREDIT CARD NO.

_____
EXPIRY DATE

_____
SIGNATURE

☐ Please invoice to above.

Publication prices will vary and are subject to change without notice. GST and Shipping & Handling Charges will be added to the invoice.